Acknowledgment

I want to thank my incredible sons, Ryan and Nick for their continuing love and support. This book would not be the same without them.

Re-Introduction

Well, it's been ten years since I wrote this book, and it has been a roller coaster ride of trying to eat raw and being tempted by the foods that smell so good when they're cooking.

In the middle of it all, I woke up one morning and thought to myself, "I don't feel good – in fact I feel horrible". It was time to take a look at my current way of eating and start to come back to foods that are fresher and provide the enzymes, nutrition and well-being that I needed.

I started juicing, eating more salads and within a couple of weeks, I was eating about 95% of my food raw. I didn't take long before I was feeling more comfortable in my body, happier, energetic and positive. I realized that going 100% raw just didn't suit me now. I eat some cooked grains (especially quinoa which is a complete protein); salad dressing at a restaurant; seared tuna; a few cooked veggies; and several other non-raw foods. I don't eat meat, pasteurized dairy, junk foods, anything artificial or fried foods. I feel clear and excited to be alive again!

I have also added some recipes that are not 100% raw, but healthy just the same. My favorite new recipe is the Cacaoballs. I just can't live without them!

My goal is to help others to see the benefit in at least going 50% raw, get rid of the fried food, junk food, and anything else that's not in it's natural state, and notice how much better they feel. I also want people who wouldn't typically think of raw foods as a way to health to consider trying it.

It hasn't been easy, but it's easier to eat this way than to deal with a host of physical ailments and the money it costs to get better.

I hope that you can make it through that first miserable couple of months and find the well being that raw food provides. An added benefit is that it raises your vibration so that life becomes easier and good things seem to come into your life as a result of feeling better. The Law of Attraction in action!

The following is the story that I wrote when I was really sick. I still believe everything; I'm just not as strict as I used to be. Whether you go 100% raw or 50% raw, I promise you that you will feel better and better as time goes on. The trick is to get a well-rounded diet of as many foods as you can, and to get the nutrition that your body needs. Have fun with it, and as you put food into your mouth, think if it will make you feel good, or make you feel bad. Think of food as a way to feel as good as you possibly can. You may find that you naturally lose weight if you're overweight, or gain weight if you're underweight. It all depends on your natural body state. Watch your eyes become clearer with more color and your skin become incredibly soft. And you won't need to worry about body odor (unless you are in the beginning detox stages).

Good luck!

2003

This is a story of getting well and becoming healthy and vibrant. **It is my story – my experience of learning and healing.** I have included instructions so that, if you choose, you can get started eating this way yourself. I hope you will find the information valuable, and that you are inspired to try raw foods and a healthy lifestyle. I've included my favorite recipes to get you started in introducing more raw foods into your eating. If you want more technical advice there are many great books available.

Why I Started Eating Raw Food

My grandfather and grandmother owned a dairy business. My grandfather died of an aneurysm and my grandmother of a heart attack, both diet related afflictions. By the time my father died of an aneurysm, he had already suffered five heart attacks and had quadruple bypass surgery. He also suffered from gout, high blood pressure, blindness and depression. His brothers all had various diet and lifestyle related ailments that can be attributed to an animal fat and protein-laden diet and unhealthy lifestyles.

I remember always being sick. When I was little, I was cold all the time. I have seen pictures of myself and my brothers swimming in the middle of summer and my lips were blue. There were times when I didn't have the energy to get out of a chair. I had earaches that would make me scream for hours. I had severe chronic fatigue syndrome in my 20's that lasted for more than two years – and I probably suffered from lingering effects until I started eating raw food. The only time I can remember feeling good in my younger years is when I decided to lose weight and quit eating for 2 weeks. I felt fantastic! And then when I started eating again, I felt horrible. I believe I had probably cleaned out my system, but started back on the wrong kinds of foods – putting new toxins in my nice clean system. That can be worse than not fasting at all. I didn't think of what I had done as fasting, and I didn't know that you should come out of a fast with good healthy foods. I came out of it eating mom's home cooking - the typical Standard American Diet (SAD) with a lot of dairy, eggs and meat; over-cooked vegetables and canned foods.

Before I started eating raw foods, I had been suffering for years from a variety of ailments: muscle twitching/cramping/numbness; numerous food allergies; tightness around my abdomen; respiratory problems; double vision; nausea; low energy; anxiety; and depression. I also experienced what felt like electrical surges through my body that would literally make me sit up in bed. Twice, I went to the hospital with symptoms of a heart attack.

I had tried a multitude of alternative practitioners, including chiropractors, acupuncturists, naturopaths, energy workers, massage therapists and more, and some would offer temporary relief, but nothing worked permanently. I was terrified and I felt frustrated and defeated. I was afraid of becoming disabled and not being able to take care of myself and dying a premature death.

I was at the end of my rope, and decided to meditate and seek an answer (something that I hadn't done often). It came to me to go to the local bookstore and take the first book off the shelf that called to me. That evening I went to the bookstore and the first book I was drawn to was Paul Nison's "Raw Knowledge". I didn't have any idea what it was about, and I wasn't familiar with raw foods, but I opened the book and read testimonials about people who live raw food lifestyles. The people looked so vibrant, healthy and young for their age that I was intrigued. I bought the book, and after bringing it home, I indulged myself in the stories for about two days. I believe now that that meditation had the perfect message for me, one that would move me farther than anything else in my life!

I decided to try raw foods and a change in lifestyle. Something inside me knew what I needed. I ate raw foods for about two weeks, and then we cooked a pizza and it was all over. The pizza smelled so good and I thought I could have just one little piece and then go back to the raw food way of eating. It didn't work - I was back to eating my typical "healthy" cooked diet. As far back as I can remember I have been conscientious about eating healthy, organic food, although almost all of it was cooked. I also ate plenty of meat. At the time it was just too hard to eat raw food when no one I knew was doing it. I was also experiencing some female hormonal problems that made me extremely weak and tired. I didn't think much about raw foods for a couple of months, but my first experience stayed in the back of my mind.

Two months went by, and I found a lump in my breast. Even with all my other symptoms, I had not seen a medical doctor because I was afraid of what they might tell me. I didn't want to be defined by some chronic, incurable disease. When I found the lump, I went to the clinic and the nurse told me she was more concerned about the lump in my other breast! She said it felt "large" and "attached". I was frightened because of the potential side effects from traditional cancer treatments; I opted instead to treat myself naturally, as naturally as I possible could. I became completely committed to eating raw foods, and living a healthy lifestyle.

A few weeks after starting on raw foods, I was still feeling the stress from the years of physical distress that I had experienced. I had to learn how to relax again, so I started doing yoga and relaxing meditations, and they helped immensely. Before starting the raw food lifestyle (notice I said lifestyle, not diet) I couldn't exercise because my muscles would cramp, ache and twitch, and I couldn't sleep. I can exercise now without a problem. I also could not eat beef, pork, fish, poultry, eggs, vinegar or soy sauce, for the same reasons. I also had a condition that prevented me from eating foods high in sulfur, such as cabbage and onions because I would feel poisoned and suffer for a couple of days. I can eat them now without any ill effect. My allergies were too numerous to mention.

I also tried colon hydrotherapy to clean out the old wastes that had accumulated in my system, to allow my digestive system to absorb more nutrients and to increase my ability to make Vitamin B12.

I'm 51 now and I feel fabulous! My skin is smoother, my hair is shinier, I have lost all the extra weight that I gained when I couldn't exercise and I'm told I look at least 10 years younger! I achieved all of this by just eating raw food until I was satisfied. It was easy! I sleep better, I handle stress better, my digestion is better, I'm free of the constipation that has plagued me for most of my life, I have more energy and my mind feels clearer. I'm just happier!

What I Eat

I had to learn a new way of thinking about food. I love food, and I loved to cook. Hot soups on a winter day were heavenly, and going to restaurants was fun. I had to think of food as nutrition and health, rather than something to comfort me, or to feed an emotion. It was very difficult at first. But now, the food I prepare is so beautiful, and so nutritionally dense, that it's easy.

When I first started eating raw foods, I was eating a lot of nuts. It seemed to give me the fullness that I desired. I ended up getting canker sores in my mouth and had to cut down. They don't bother me at all anymore. I'm not sure why that has changed. It may be that the pH level in my body is more alkaline. Another thing that I initially had to deal with was gas and bloating, but I found that if I didn't eat fruits (except apples), and vegetables at the same meal, and I cut down on the amount of food I ate at a sitting, it wasn't serious. Some of the raw food books can be very strict about food combinations but that's not a great concern to me. I love food and I love variety at a meal. Now, if I get a little bloated, it's gone the next day. I don't think I could eat this way if I was too strict.

To sweeten food, I use only agave nectar, honey, maple syrup, dates, raisins, and figs. Other dried fruits such as prunes, apricots along with many fresh fruits can be used to sweeten food as well. I would recommend staying away from all concentrated sweeteners such as sugar and corn syrup. Some people use Stevia, but it has a taste some don't like.

One of my staples is my Creamy Tahini Dressing. I use it on many different salads. Another favorite condiment is Eden's Seaweed Gomasio. It doesn't have a fishy flavor, so if you don't like seaweed, it's a good way to get the value from seaweed without the taste.

I have also included Spirulina in my diet, as it provides chlorophyll, which is a nutrient-rich food for cellular health and high energy. It provides antioxidants, carotenoids and phytonutrients. Spirulina has also been found to support a healthy immune system.

BASICS OF GOOD NUTRITION

Why Raw?

Why raw foods? …Because that's what we were meant to eat. It's very simple. Our bodies are not meant to eat animal products, or cooked food. Cooking vegetables denatures them, and takes out valuable vitamins and minerals. I have heard people say that eating raw vegetables is hard on the digestive tract, and you may find some discomfort at first, but my experience is that it's easier than eating cooked foods. My digestion has never been better. It's all so simple, but we've come a long way from our natural way of eating. And we have great memories of homemade stew, turkey dinners, meatloaf, barbequed chicken, etc. They all taste so good (at least they used to). We relate to food through our memories. If we had never eaten cooked food in our life, we wouldn't be attached to it. Cooked food is addictive. I didn't believe it at first but now I am a believer. The first two weeks without cooked food were awful. Every time I smelled pizza, or drove by a place cooking hamburgers, I would salivate and my taste buds would go wild. I felt like Pavlov's dog. I had dreams at night of Kentucky Fried Chicken and Big Macs even though I had not tasted either for at least 15 years. It's easy to go a couple of weeks without a salad, carrot or an apple. But try going a couple of weeks without cooked food and see what happens. You'll be as amazed as I was at what your body, mind and emotions go through.

Nutrition

I had the typical concerns that people have about eating this way. "How will I get protein, Vitamin B12, and calcium?" I thought they weren't significant in raw foods. And then the more I read and studied; I came to a whole new understanding of how our bodies work in relation to food. How does a gorilla, a cow, or a giraffe get the protein to create those big muscular bodies? Protein is built from amino acids, which are available in fruits, vegetables, nuts, seeds, legumes and grains. The truth about food and what we have been taught are two very different things. Regarding dairy – I believe we need much less calcium than the dairy industry claims we do, and we can get it from green leafy vegetables. All the nutrients we need are in raw and living foods. And the healthier we are, the better our bodies assimilate these nutrients. Vitamin B12 is made in abundance in a healthy digestive system, and we can get it in certain sprouts in a very useable form.

Roe Gallo comments in *Perfect Body*, "Imagine yourself on an island full of beautiful fruit trees, lush grasses, animals, birds, insects, fish and other creatures. Imagine that you get hungry. What would you be most inclined to eat? Would you rip into a cow, a pig, a bird, or fish…. Or, would you pick a mouthwatering, sugar-sweet luscious fruit from one of the trees?" The fruit tree would be our natural choice of food of course (at least I hope). We are the only species on earth that eats things that are not appealing to us in their natural state. A cow just isn't appealing to human beings. Its not even appealing cut up in pieces in the supermarket. It's not until it's cooked that it becomes appealing, and when you have been on a raw food diet for a while, it's not even appealing then. I can't even imagine looking at a chicken and thinking "food". I have a hard time looking at or even smelling the raw meat in the supermarket now. It's just doesn't look natural, and I can smell the bacteria. Natural foods appeal to our senses in their natural state. They look great, smell great and they taste great. And we feel so good when we eat them.

A distinction that I think is important when eating this way is between raw and living foods. A living food is a freshly picked fruit or vegetable (within 24 hours), or sprouted nuts/seeds/grains/legumes with all of the enzymes and nutrients still intact. Raw foods are those that are uncooked. The natural enzymes that are missing in the Standard American

Diet are available in raw and living foods - more in living foods. When you eat raw foods, you won't feel the typical heaviness of the Standard American Diet. You will have to grow accustomed to feeling lighter. But over time you will notice that you need less and less food to feel full. You are getting so many more nutrients, that you don't need the quantities that you needed before. In fact I've noticed that I enjoy eating like this so much, that I wish I could just eat all day, but my stomach won't let me. And you can be assured that if you are eating various fruits, vegetables, nuts, grains, sprouts, legumes and raw cheeses that you are getting what you need.

Support

I think it's important to have support either through books, friends, family or people that are raw foodists, while you are beginning this way of eating. It is not a common way to eat, although right now it is among the top 7 diets in popularity. I didn't know anyone who was doing it when I started. I live in a city where more people eat Jell-O and Ice Cream per capita than anywhere else in the world. I had to read a number of raw food related books, and testimonials on the Internet to stay inspired. And of course the lumps in my breasts were the biggest motivator. Once I started to feel and look great, that was my motivation. Then I met a man who was giving raw food demonstrations at a health food store near my home. It was so exciting to meet someone else who believed in this way of life. He was so alive, healthy and happy. His eyes sparkled, and he loved life. He was very inspiring. He now owns "Omar's Rawtopia Restaurant" in Salt Lake City, Utah. Check it out if you're there. It has great food. Another thing is to check to see if they are offering any raw food events in your area. A good Internet sight is Living Nutrition at http://www.livingnutrition.com. They have an abundance of information on raw food - including a magazine, books, events, products, recipes, connections, counseling and testimonials. Another sight is Raw Foods at http://www.rawfood.com/. Now I have found a couple of local monthly raw food potlucks that have the nicest people and the greatest food. It's fun to share my story and hear other people's stories of miraculous healings including cancer and childhood diabetes.

When I speak to people of this way of eating, I see a glimmer in their eyes, and they are genuinely interested. I think somewhere in our subconscious we know that it is the perfect way to eat. Especially interested are the people who know me and see how I've transformed. Some of my friends and family have even introduced more raw foods and juices into their way of eating. Sticking to it isn't easy. There are so many temptations out there. The smell of restaurants, the dinner parties, the social aspect, memories of your comfort foods, family members cooking food, having to cook for someone else, traveling - are all temptations. And when your body starts to detox and you don't feel good, it's really easy to want to go back to your old way of eating. That's when, if you stick it out, you will just keep feeling better and better. I understand that it's not easy, especially if you are experiencing headaches, diarrhea, or any of the other common detox symptoms. But if you give it a couple of months, you will notice such differences in the way you feel and look that you will want to stay with it. A month isn't very long – try it and see.

Exercise

As we all know, another aspect of good health is exercise. But I couldn't exercise for so long, that I had to work into it gradually. If you are out of shape, it's difficult to develop a lifestyle of constant exercise but it is essential. Exercise contributes so much to our overall attitude and carriage. I had the posture of someone who felt beaten down in life. Now I notice myself sitting up straight and walking taller.

Positive Attitude

A positive attitude is essential to good health but sometimes it just isn't very easy. In the beginning whenever I tried to think positively, my mind would get more and more negative. I had to let my mind do what it was going to do, and fill it with positive, inspirational messages; meditate; get fresh air; sunshine; exercise; and of course raw nutrient dense food. Over time I automatically became more positive. I don't know what it is about raw food, but it really helped with my thinking. Maybe the life in the food made me feel more alive and more positive. I was an anxious person, but since I have changed my lifestyle, I feel much more calm, relaxed and happy.

Water

Drinking water is another important aspect of good health. There is a lot of conflicting information about the type of water to drink. I started out drinking distilled water, but it is quite costly to buy, so I switched to filtered water that I refill at the health food store. Whichever you choose, they are both better than tap water, which has high concentrations of chlorine and other chemicals. You will want to drink a lot of water at first when your body is detoxing. Detoxification can appear as a number of physical, mental and emotional symptoms. My symptoms were like a very strong cold. I had a lot of phlegm, and felt cold and shivery with low energy. You may experience some of the other common detoxification symptoms that I have already mentioned. Water will help remove the toxins from your body quickly. A little lemon in your water first thing in the morning is good for the kidneys and liver. "CELLFOOD" by NuScience is also a great addition to your drinking water. It contains 78 minerals, 34 enzymes, and 17 amino acids. It provides a powerful stream of bio-available oxygen plus 129 nutrients directly to the cells. It can be found at http://www.cellfood.com/.

THE RAW FOOD LIFESTYLE

Transitioning to Raw Foods

When you are transitioning from the Standard American Diet to the raw foods lifestyle, you may feel that you need more foods with fat in them, such as nuts or avocados in order to get the feeling of fullness that you're accustomed to. I say do whatever you need initially to get you through the transition. In the beginning, I was eating a lot of avocados and nuts, and a good portion of pie every few days (and I began losing weight!) If you need to make a pie every day, or dehydrated cookies – do so until you get to the point where those things are more of a treat than part of your everyday nutrition. And then start eating more fruits, vegetables and sprouts as you become accustomed to this way of eating.

Dehydrating

Sometimes it's hard to eat cold food if it's cold outside, and you are just starting out. A good way to satisfy that feeling of warmth is to dehydrate food or set it in the sun for an hour or two. When I first started, it was December, and I would think about cooked foods constantly. At first I did a lot of dehydrated food and hot herbal teas just to experience some warmth.

Dehydrating raw food is especially good during the transition phase. You may miss a few nutrients, but you keep the live enzymes intact that are so important. You can make cookies, crackers, nut loaves, burgers and even pizza! They provide warmth and a satisfying texture. Allowing the temperature of the food to exceed 118 degrees will kill the enzymes that are so important to your health. When that happens, your body has to borrow enzymes to assimilate the food and over time you end up with a negative balance in your body and tissue begins to break down. The definition of an enzyme is: "any of various complex organic substances originating from living cells and capable of producing by catalytic action certain chemical changes in organic substances." If your body doesn't have the enzymes it needs to break food down, your body will suffer. You can use a dehydrator to dry vegetables, fruits and herbs during fall harvest to prepare for winter months. In the summer you can use the sun to dehydrate foods by placing them on a screen with airflow above and below.

Juicing

Juicing is a good way to transition into raw foods. If you haven't eaten much raw food, and you want the benefits of raw fruits and vegetables in concentrated form, start juicing every day. Carrot and apple juice are typically the best tasting at first. You can add other veggies as you become accustomed to juicing. Green vegetable juices are very cleansing. I don't really like the taste of green juices, even though I know they're very good for me. My favorite is carrot, apple, celery and ginger. Whatever you do, make it pleasant and fun so you stick with it.

Sprouts

Sprouting is essential to a nutritional way of eating, especially if you have cold winters and fresh fruits and veggies are not available. Sprouts contain the highest source of active enzymes of all foods as well as the best forms of vitamins and minerals. They are easier to assimilate than any other food source, and they can even help repair DNA and RNA. According to Gabriel Cousins, M.D., research suggests that enzymes balance and enhance the immune system, help to heal cancer, multiple sclerosis, scurvy, rheumatoid diseases and arthritis. I always have several types of sprouts growing. They are very easy to produce. Just take a quart glass jar and put the seed, grain or legume in the jar with water to cover and leave overnight. The sprouts are going to expand greatly so take that into consideration when deciding the quantity. In the morning, attach cheesecloth over the opening of the jar secured by a rubber band. Pour off the water, rinse and invert into a bowl at about a 45-degree angle. I use a wooden dish drainer with a towel underneath, but you can simply use a bowl if you like. Rinse twice a day, and when your seeds have sprouted to the length that you like, let them sit in the sun for about 6 hours to develop chlorophyll and then store in the refrigerator. Some of the sprouts I like are: lentils, which contain vitamins C, E, B-12, and are rich in iron and complete protein; mung beans (my favorite); which contain vitamins C, E, B-12, protein, iron and potassium sunflower seeds; quinoa; radish (spicy) and fenugreek, probably the most medicinal of all of the sprouts. Fenugreek has been reported to be a cure for just about everything. Some other choices are: alfalfa; turnip; onion; garlic; kale; cabbage; celery; chia; amaranth; red clover; arugula; fennel; broccoli; mustard; chick peas; adzuki beans, lima beans; pinto beans; northern white beans; green peas; triticale, wheat, millet; spelt; rye; barley; teff; quinoa; sesame seeds; sunflower seeds; pumpkin seeds; corn; and wild rice. There are many good sources on the internet for ordering sprouting seeds with recipes, sprouting kits, and additional sprouting information.

Some of the ways to use sprouts are:

- Just the way they are in salads
- Grains for sprouted, dehydrated bread
- Grind and add to crackers before dehydrating
- Add to smoothies
- Juice with things such as apples or carrots
- Use in soups or as toppings for soups
- Sprinkle around an entrée for a nice garnish
- Eat them as a snack – like popcorn
- Put them in sandwiches

The Hippocrates Health Institute in West Palm Beach, Florida helps people cleanse and detoxify their bodies and take control of their health. They are great supporters of sprouts in every way shape or form. The following benefits of sprouts is taken from their book *"Living Foods for Optimum Health"* with some additional information from Wikipedia and the Sprout People (http://www.sproutpeople.com):

Buckwheat: Good source of lecithin for lowering cholesterol, promoting weight loss, and supporting liver health. Best at 1/8".

Pumpkin: Good source of Protein, Iron, Zinc, Manganese, Magnesium, Phosphorus, Copper, and Potassium. They also provide Polyunsaturated Fatty Acids (including the essential fatty acids Omega-3 and Omega-6), which are good for the skin and hair. Best at 1/8".

Sesame: Good source of Calcium. They also contain Vitamins B, C and E, Iron, Magnesium, Pantothenic Acid, Phosphorus, Amino Acids, and Protein: 15%. Best at 1/8"

Sunflower: Good for Protein and Energy. Best at ½".

Amaranth: Good for strengthening the bones. Best at 1/8".

Millet: The Protein content in millet is very close to that of wheat; both provide about 11% Protein by weight. It is rich in B Vitamins, especially Niacin, B6 and Folic Acid,

Calcium, Iron, Potassium, Magnesium, and Zinc, which makes it good for Strength and Muscle. Best at 1/8".

Quinoa: High Protein content: 12-18%, and a balanced set of Amino Acids making it a complete protein source. High in Fiber, Magnesium and Iron. Good for Strength and Energy. Best at ¼".

Teff: Very high calcium content, and high levels of Phosphorus, Iron, Copper, Aluminum, Barium, and Thiamin. The Iron from teff is easily absorbed by the body, which is a big advantage. Teff is high in Protein. Good for Blood and Respiration. Best at 1/8"

Barley: Good source of Protein, Thiamine, Niacin, Vitamin B6, Iron, Magnesium, Phosphorous, and Zinc. It is good for the ventricles and heart. Best when just soaked and not sprouted.

Corn: Has significant Antioxidant activity. Good for Calcium and Energy. Best at ½".

Spelt: Vitamins and Minerals. Best at ¼".

Triticale: Calcium, Vitamins and Minerals. Best at ¼".

Wheat: Vitamins and Minerals. Good for making Rejuvalac. Best at ¼".

Adzuki Beans: Minerals and renal benefits. Best at 1".

Chickpeas: Good source of Zinc, Folate and Protein. They are also very high in Dietary Fiber. Good for Protein and Energy. Best at 1".

Lentils: High levels of Proteins, including all of the Essential Amino Acids. They also include Dietary Fiber, Folate, Vitamin B1, and Minerals. Good for Teeth and Strength. Best at 1".

Green Peas: Vitamins A, B, C and E, Calcium, Iron, Phosphorus, Amino Acids, Protein: 25%. Good for Blood and Organs. Best at 1".

Lima Beans: Lima beans have the Trace Mineral, Molybdenum, an integral component of the enzyme sulfite oxidase, and it detoxifies sulfites. Good for the Nails and Eyes. Best when soaked and not sprouted.

Mung Beans: Good source of Phosphorous, Vitamins A, B, C and E, Calcium, Iron, Magnesium, Potassium, Amino

Acids, and Protein: 20%. Also has Bladder Benefits. Good in Asian dishes. Best at 1/8" to 2" depending on what you're using them for. I like them when they just begin to show a sprout. They are sweet and you can eat as a snack.

Northern White Beans: High in Protein and Dietary Fiber and is an excellent source of Iron, Potassium, Selenium, Molybdenum, Thiamine, Vitamin B6, and Folic Acid. Good for Energy and the Liver. Best when just soaked and not sprouted.

Pinto Beans: High in Protein and Dietary Fiber and is an excellent source of Pantothenic Acid, Folate, Calcium, Iron, Magnesium and Zinc. Good for Energy and the Spine. Best at 1".

Alfalfa: Probably the most popular of all the sprouts. They are a good source of Vitamins A, B, C, E and K Calcium, Iron, Magnesium, Phosphorus, Potassium, Zinc, Carotene, Chlorophyll, Amino Acids, Trace Elements, Protein: 35%. Good for the Blood and the Heart. Best at 2".

Cabbage: Vitamins A, B, C, E and K, Calcium, Iron, Magnesium, Phosphorus, Potassium, Zinc, Carotene, Chlorophyll, Amino Acids, Trace Elements, Antioxidants, Protein: 35%. Good for the Intestines and the Stomach. Best at 1 ½".

Clover: Vitamins A, B, C, E and K, Calcium, Iron, Magnesium, Phosphorus, Potassium, Zinc, Carotene, Chlorophyll, Amino Acids, Trace Elements, Protein: 35%. Good for Capillaries and the Blood. Excellent for Women. Best at 2".

Fenugreek: Vitamins A, B, C, E, Calcium, Iron, Magnesium, Phosphorus, Potassium, Zinc, Carotene, Chlorophyll, Phyto-Nutrients - Excellent for Women (Breast Health), Amino Acids, Trace Elements, Digestive Aid, Protein: 30%. Dissolves mucous and deposits. Best at 2".

Garlic: Vitamins A, B, C, and E, Calcium, Iron, Magnesium, Phosphorus, Potassium, Zinc, Carotene,

Chlorophyll, Amino Acids, Trace Elements, Protein: 20%. Good for the Heart and Cholesterol. Best at 1".

Kale: Kale is considered to be a highly nutritious vegetable with powerful antioxidant properties and is anti-inflammatory. Kale is very high in Beta Carotene, Vitamin K, Vitamin C, Lutein, Zeaxanthin, and reasonably rich in Calcium. They are good to use as micro greens, (instructions follow) and then use as beautiful garnishes on a plate. Because of its high vitamin K content, patients taking anti-coagulants such as warfarin are encouraged to avoid this food since it increases the vitamin K concentration in the blood, which is what the drugs are often attempting to lower. This effectively raises the effective dose of the drug. They are good for the bowels. Best at 1".

Mustard: Vitamins A, B, C, E and K, Calcium, Iron, Magnesium, Phosphorus, Potassium, Zinc, Carotene, Chlorophyll, Amino Acids, Trace Elements, Antioxidants, Protein: 35% Tastes like horseradish. Good for the Stomach and Gall Bladder. Best at 1 ½".

Onion: Vitamins A, B, C, E and K, Calcium, Iron, Magnesium, Phosphorus, Potassium, Zinc, Carotene, Chlorophyll, Amino Acids, Trace Elements, Antioxidants, Protein: 20%. Taste just like onions. Good for the Blood and Circulation. Best at 1 ½".

Radish: Rich in Ascorbic Acid, Folic Acid, and Potassium. They are a good source of Vitamin B6, Riboflavin, Magnesium, Copper, and Calcium. They are good for the Lymph and Hormones. Best at 2".

Turnip: High in Vitamin C, Vitamin A, Folate, Vitamin C, Vitamin K, Calcium, and Lutein. Good for the Colon and Intestine. Best at 1 ½".

Wheatgrass

Wheatgrass has massive amounts of chlorophyll. It is similar to the structure of human red blood cells, which helps the blood's capacity to carry oxygen throughout the body. It can also neutralize toxins in the body. It also helps cleanse the body and rebuild cells.

I have a difficult time drinking wheatgrass. I don't like the taste, and it can cause nausea if you have a lot of toxins in your system.

I prefer to get my nutrition from the myriad other available sprouts that are easy to eat and sprout. Some people may find therapeutic uses for wheatgrass, though, such as treating a peptic ulcer and ulcerative colitis.

Micro Greens can be used like sprouts. They are like miniature plants that are great in any dish where you use sprouts. They also make beautiful garnishes.

Sprouting Instructions for Micro Greens:

- Soak for about 8-12 hours prior to sprouting in cool water. Drain (use water to water your houseplants if you like).
- Rinse thoroughly in cool water. Drain thoroughly.
- Place a paper towel on your sprouting tray to retain moisture. Pour the seeds onto the paper towel and rinse once a day for a couple of days. Place out of direct sunlight. You want 1/16 to 1/8 inch roots.
- Plant in a tray with soil or planting medium. Spread seeds so that they each have space to grow.
- Water or mist every day or two. You want them to be moist, but not soggy.
- When they start to shed there hulls, put them in full sunlight.
- When your plants have open, green leaves, they are done.
- Harvest by cutting just above the soil.
- Store dry plants in the refrigerator until ready to use.

You can also grow your micro greens in something called a Miniature Garden from the Sprout People, or you can get creative and grow them on fabric or a paper towel!

Just imagine if you ate a variety of sprouts and micro greens every day how great you would feel!

Edible Flowers

The following is a list of edible, common flowers that you can add to your salads or sandwiches to make them more nutritious and beautiful. They also make beautiful, edible garnishes.

Bachelor's Buttons	Mint
Basil	Mustard
Borage	Nasturtium
Broccoli	Orange Blossom
Calendula	Oregano
Carnation	Pansy
Catnip	Pea
Chamomile	Peppermint
Chive	Pinks
Cilantro	Radish
Dandelion	Red Clover
Dill	Rose (not commercial
Fennel	varieties as they contain
Gardenia	many pesticides)
Garlic	Rosemary
Garlic Chive	Sage
Hibiscus	Spearmint
Honeysuckle	Squash
Hyssop	Sunflower
Jasmine	Thyme
Johnny-Jump-Up	Tulip
Kale	Violet
Lavender	Watercress
Lemon	Yarrow
Lemon Balm	Yucca
Marjoram	

Cultured Food

What is a cultured food?

Cultured food means food that is created out of the interaction between beneficial flora and a food source. Cultured food does most of the digestive work for us and makes the nutrients more bioavailable and also enhances our immune system. The lactobacillus that is created by fermentation helps to break down sugars and starches, which help aid in proper digestion. If you have ever taken antibiotics and have not replaced these helpful little lactobacilli bacteria, you could have problems down the line.

Some of the ways that people culture foods is by making kefir, yogurt, miso, or culturing vegetables. If you are making your own kefir and yogurt, it is best to use raw milks. Kefir can also be made from the milk of the young green coconut. A great how-to book for making kefir is *Body Ecology* by Donna Gates. It also has additional information on cultured foods in general. You can find more information on her website: http://www.bodyecology.com/.

Miso can be purchased pretty much anywhere, including typical grocery stores. It is not raw, but is considered part of a raw food diet because it contains all of the enzymes found in raw food. If you cannot find it in your area, there are a number of online companies to order from.

Cultured foods have really helped my digestive system. They are tasty to boot. I add them to salads and eat them just as they are.

Unfortunately, the commercial sauerkraut that you find bottled in stores has been pasteurized and the healthy enzymes have been destroyed.

Rejuvenative Foods sell a variety of healthy, organic, raw, cultured vegetables. You can find them at: http://www.rejuvenative.com.

Other cultured foods include Kefir and Kombucha. You can read more about cultured foods at: http://culturedfoodlife.com/.

Sea Vegetables

The mineral content of sea vegetables or seaweeds is extraordinary. All of the common edible seaweeds are higher in vitamins and trace minerals than any land vegetable, including vitamins A, B1, B2, B6, B12, C, Niacin, Potassium, Magnesium and Calcium. A great number of organic compounds known as phyto (plant) chemicals are found in sea vegetables. Many of these organic compounds are necessary, but missing in our modern food supply. Sea vegetables are very alkaline and a diet rich in alkalinizing plant foods has shown to help preserve muscle mass in older men and women. Seaweed has essential fatty acids, nucleic acids like RNA and DNA, phyto-chemicals as carotenoids (anti oxidants), protein and fiber. They are also virtually fat-free and a low calorie food.

The benefits of including seaweed's optimum nourishment into your daily diet are extensive: increased longevity, enhanced immune functioning, revitalization of the cardiovascular, endocrine, digestive, and nervous systems, and relief from minor aches and pains.

Nori is the most common seaweed as it is used to wrap sushi. It aids in digestion and colon cleansing.

Arame has a mild sweet taste.

Wakame has a delicate texture and flavor.

Hijiki is stronger tasting and somewhat crunchy.

Sea Lettuce is tender and used in soups and sandwiches. It resembles lettuce.

Dulse has a mild texture and strong flavor. It is usually ground and added to dishes.

Bladderwrack and **Kelp** are high in good phytoestrogens, which promote healthy breast tissue.

Kombu has high concentrations of Iodine, which pulls radiation, as well as other heavy metals out of the human body. It also works with the pancreas to break down lipids.

Irish Rockweed can be used in weight-loss.

Superfoods

There is a fairly new category of foods called superfoods.
These are foods that have a high nutritional or health benefit
that are not common to the foods we typically eat everyday. It
is hard to say what a superfood really is, because there are so
many foods that are beneficial to us.

David Wolfe on his Sunfood Nutrition website lists Aloe Vera,
Bee Pollen, Blue-Green Algae, Cacao, Camu Camu, Goji
Berries, Green Superfood, Maca, Medicinal Mushrooms, Noni,
Rice Protein, and Sea Vegetables as superfoods. If I were to
list a few more they would be Spirulina, Coconut Butter, Raw
Honey and Acai.

Try some of the superfoods and see how you feel. I like Maca,
Sea Vegetables, Spirulina, Coconut Butter and Raw Honey.
I've never heard of Camu Camu before. I read that it contains
more Vitamin C than any other known botanical source and
comes from the South American Rain Forest.

A lot of raw foods can now be ordered on EBay and you can
save quite a bit of money ordering that way.

Cacao

I have a whole section devoted to cacao because I think the
benefits are many.

Studies indicate that the antioxidants in cacao can prevent the
oxidation of LDL-cholesterol, related to the protection in heart
disease. Cacao may even help lower hypertension and may be
beneficial in Alzheimer's prevention.

Eating cacao may help lower blood pressure, boost normal
responses to insulin to keep blood sugar levels down, and
improve blood vessel function in patients with high blood
pressure, according to new research findings. These could cut

the risk of heart attack and stroke and possibly prevent hardening of arteries

Early records indicate that cacao was used as a medicine. It was known to improve digestion and stimulate kidney and bowel function. Additional diseases that responded to treatment using cacao were anemia, fatigue, fever, low sex drive, respiratory troubles, poor appetite and low breast milk production. In addition to the cacao bean, the oil/butter was used in the treatment of skin problems including eczema, psoriasis and burns.

Cacoa has tryptophan - an anti-depressant, arginine – a natural aphrodisiac and other beneficial compounds known to have rejuvenating and anti-aging effects.

Cacao is especially high in magnesium which is responsible for a number of benefits including it's calming qualities, heart health, bone health, and keeping blood pressure low. It also contains sulphur, which is good for the health of the skin, nails and hair.

Buy Organic

Try to buy organic food whenever possible. When you are taking such great care of your body by eating raw food, it makes sense to keep as many toxins out of your body as possible. You can buy organic food at health food stores, Asian markets, on the Internet, local farms and farmers markets. The ideal way to eat organic food is freshly picked right from your own garden. It has the most nutrient value, and you know that it is 100% organic. If you don't have much room, you can grow vegetables and herbs in containers outside, or plant them throughout your flower garden if you have one.

Tools

Two of the most important tools that you will use when preparing raw foods are a blender and a food processor. The blender is good for making salad dressing and smoothies, and the food processor is used for most food preparation. I use it everyday. A juicer is an excellent piece of equipment. A dehydrator will become a mini replacement for your oven. A coffee grinder is useful for grinding herbs, spices and seeds. Flax meal is something that you may use quite a bit, and a coffee grinder does a great job of grinding it into a fine meal. I also use it for grinding things like cumin seeds, whole nutmeg, brown mustard seed, cinnamon sticks, and cardamom. Another tool is a Spiralizer or Garnishing Machine. You can use these to make "spaghetti" out of zucchini, yams, carrots, beets, squash, etc. A nut bag is nice to have for straining the liquid from the pulp when making nut milks, although you can use cheesecloth too.

Staying Raw

Don't be surprised if you feel awful after a few weeks, and then occasionally thereafter until your body is cleansed. The raw foods are cleaning out your system. As the body is getting rid of the toxins that have accumulated over the years, people experience a variety of symptoms - headaches, lethargy, forgetfulness, nightmares, rashes, diarrhea, runny nose, coughing, and a number of other ailments. The worse you have eaten, the worse the symptoms may be. You can find yourself purging some old emotions as well. Just know that it gets better. In fact it gets amazing! As you lose the toxins in your system, you may become thinner than you would like (although I never did), but you will probably gain some weight and then stabilize at the weight you are supposed to be. I lost 20 pounds in the first four months, which brought me to my perfect weight.

When you feel that you want to go back to old habits and eat cooked food, just remember the benefits of a raw food lifestyle. Some typical benefits are: superb health, immunity from chronic illnesses; clear skin; more energy; weight loss; better hearing and eyesight; radiance; spiritual awareness; joy; higher vibration; aliveness; and on and on. I believe that the "Life" in the food gives you "Life" in your body.

Cleansing

Good cleansing of your system will happen naturally over time with a raw food diet, but there are ways to accelerate the removal of toxins and debris from your body.

Some of the cleanses that you can do once you have become accustomed to this way of eating are: colon cleanses, liver cleanses, gall bladder cleanses, liquid diets, herbal cleanses, and a myriad of other cleanses depending on your situation.

Body Brushes

Your body is the largest eliminative organ in the body and body brushing can help remove toxins from the skin and help lighten the load. It stimulates the lymphatic system and removes waste from the body. Before taking a bath or shower remove your clothes and start with your feet and move up your legs using upward strokes. You can use circular strokes in the area of cellulite (thighs and buttocks) to help remove fat stores. Brush up the torso using small strokes and avoid the breasts. If you have a brush with a long handle it helps in getting the back area. Make long strokes from your hands to your shoulders. You'll feel energized if you do this on a daily basis! It's especially great in the initial stages when you may be experiencing detox symptoms.

Making It Easy

Some ways to make raw food preparation a little easier are to keep soaked dates in the refrigerator all of the time; chop up vegetables in separate containers to add to salads, start the sprout soaking process and rinse process the same time everyday, so you don't forget; and dehydrate a lot of cookies, bars, crackers, etc. when you have the time. Things like the Nut & Veggie Burgers, Apple Cinnamon Granola, Ginger Pancakes, Lentil and Cumin Salad, Sweet & Sour Lentils, Adzuki & Wild Rice Salad, Dilled Green Beans, Salad Dressings, Hummus, Sun-Dried Olive Tepanade, Homemade Horseradish, Nut Cream Cheese, Cashew Mayonnaise, Energy Bars and Pies will all last about a week, so you can prepare them one day and have them throughout the week.
After you have been on the raw food way of living for a little while, it's easy to get a little over zealous. You're feeling so good, and you want everyone to experience what you're feeling, especially your family and close friends. But not everyone is going to feel the same about your way of eating.

The best you can do is to be an inspiration, and answer questions if they ask. I try to find out if raw food is something people want to hear about. If not, I don't push it anymore. It's easy for me if people are complaining about a health problem, to say, "just eat raw foods", but most people aren't prepared to hear that. I would rather let people find their own way, rather than risk turning them off to this life style. The best teacher is inspiration.

The recipes that follow are my favorites. You can adjust them as your tastes desire.

This is a list of staples that are good to have available, although not necessary. You can start out small and add to them over time.

Agave Nectar
Honey
Maple Syrup

Olive Oil
Dried Coconut
Coconut Butter
Vanilla Extract
Raw Tahini
Raw Almond Butter
Herbamare
Eden's Seaweed Gomasio
Sea Salt
Nama Shoyu (raw soy sauce)
Cashews
Almonds
Pecans
Sesame Seeds
Quinoa
Wild Rice
Cacao Beans, Nibs and Powder (Raw Chocolate)
Raisins
Dates
Almond Flour
Raw Cheeses
Lemons
Garlic
Frozen Peas
Fresh Veggies and Fruits
Assorted Seeds for Sprouting

Appliances that are good to have:

Food Processor
Blender
Dehydrator w/ Teflex Sheets
Nut Bag
Spiralizer
Mandolin
Juicer
Vita Mix

Replace   # With

Replace	With
Canned Tomatoes	Hydrated Sun-Dried Tomatoes
Whipping Cream	Soaked Cashews Creamed in FP
Tuna	Soaked Walnuts & Kelp
Parmesan Cheese	Raw Macadamias & Lemon Juice
Cream in Soup	Coconut Milk
Regular Cheese	Raw Cheese or Seed Cheese
Sugar	Agave Nectar/Honey/Dates/Raisins
Spaghetti Noodles	Zucchini/Yellow Squash Spiralized
White Flour	Almond Meal/Flax Meal
Canned Juices	Fresh Juices (not pasteurized)
Milk	Almond Milk (or other nut milks)
Cereal	Dehydrated Granola
Hamburgers	Nut Burgers or Veggie Burgers
White Cooked Rice	Chopped Macadamia or Pine Nuts
Regular Sushi	Vegetable Sushi
Tortillas	Dehydrated Tortillas/Chard Leaves
Cocoa Powder	Ground Cacao or Carob Powder
Bottled Chutney	Fresh Chutney
Canned Garbanzos	Sprouted Garbanzos
Typical Crackers	Whole Grain Crackers or dehydrated crackers
Roasted/Salted Nuts	Nuts soaked in Nama Shoyu and Dehydrated
Store-bought Cookies	Dehydrated Cookies
Junk Snacks	Celery/Carrot Sticks; Dates stuffed with Pecans; Air-popped Popcorn; Fresh Fruit; Fresh Fruit Smoothies
Baked Pie Crust	2 cups nuts/1 cup dates or raisins processed in food processor and pressed into pie plate
Traditional Peanut Butter	Raw nut butters from health food store
Traditional Jam or Jelly	Fruit and agave nectar processed in food Processor
Chocolate Chips	Cacao Nibs

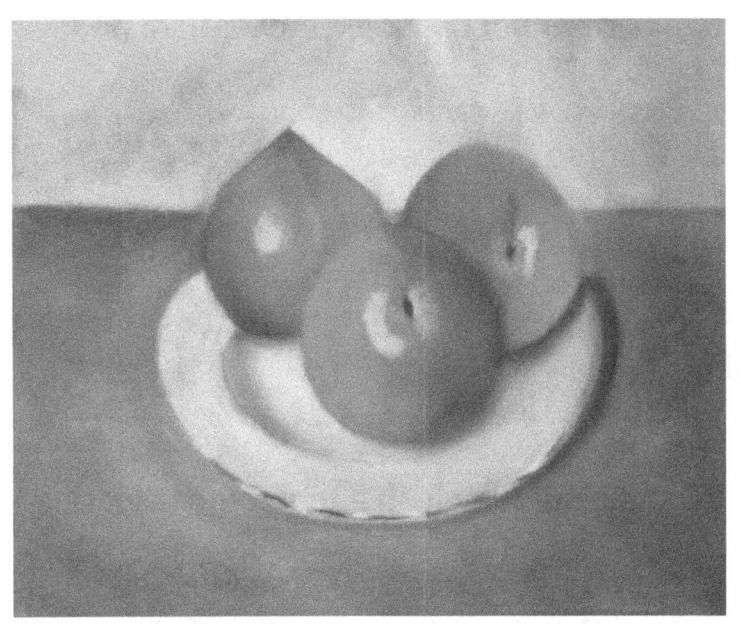

BREAKFAST

apple cinnamon granola

1 cup pecans, soaked overnight and drained
1 cup almonds, soaked overnight and drained
1 cup sunflower seeds, soaked overnight and
    drained
½ cup sesame seeds
2 apples, cored and diced
1 tsp vanilla
2 cups dates, soaked
1 cup raisins, soaked
2 Tbl cinnamon
dash salt
enough purified water to blend

Combine all ingredients in a food processor and
blend using the "S" blade until pieces are very
small. Spread mixture on Teflex sheet and
dehydrate for about 12 hours. Serve with
Homemade Almond Milk.

breakfast of champions

1 banana, sliced
½ cup mango, diced
½ cup papaya, diced
1 pear, cut in chunks
2 large dates, chopped
½ cup cashews (whole or pieces)
sprinkling of shaved coconut

Mix together in a bowl and serve. This dish will help replace the typical egg and toast breakfast. It is very filling. I eat it just about every morning.

ginger pancakes

1 tsp grated fresh ginger
1 cup cashews, soaked overnight and drained
1 cup pecans, soaked overnight and drained
1 apple, grated
½ cup flaxmeal
10 dates, soaked (save water)
½ cup date soaking water
1 tsp cinnamon
½ tsp cardamom
½ tsp vanilla

Combine all ingredients in a food processor and blend using the "S" blade. Add more date water if needed to make a thick batter. Make into 3" pancakes on a dehydrator sheet and dry for about 6 hours. Flip and dehydrate another 4 hours. Serve with fresh fruit and date syrup (water from soaking dates), agave syrup or honey.

These are not your typical fluffy pancakes. They are dense and soft – but good.

almost raw granola

1 cup cashews, soaked for 30 minutes
1 cup pecans, soaked for 30 minutes
1 1/3 cup rolled oat flakes
½ cup raisins
¼ cup maple syrup
¼ cup agave nectar
¼ cup melted organic butter
dash cinnamon & nutmeg
dash salt

Drain and chop the cashews and pecans. Mix together the nuts, oat flakes and raisins. Combine the maple syrup, agave nectar, butter, cinnamon, nutmeg and salt. Pour over the oat mixture and dehydrate on Teflex sheets about 12 hours at 115 degrees.

You can add chopped apricots, bananas, apples, almonds or anything you like.

spirulina pudding blast

meat from one young green coconut
1 Tbl powdered spirulina
1 Tbl hemp seeds
2 Tbl Really Raw Honey©*

Combine ingredients in a blender or Vita Mix. Prepare to be blasted with energy.

You can add cacao powder; soaked chia seeds; substitute a dash of Stevia for the honey; or anything else your heart desires.

*I use *Really Raw Honey©* which is a brand that doesn't use any heat in preparing the honey. It won't ever get sugary and hard like honey that has been heated. It's creamy and wonderful. It makes all the difference. Some companies say their honey is raw, because they use low heat to remove the honey from the comb and it still has the enzymes, but if it is runny at all, it has been heated and just won't taste the same.

Really Raw Honey© can be found at http://www.reallyrawhoney.com/.

breakfast smoothie

meat and water from one young green coconut
2 bananas
10 dates (soaked for at least 4 hours) along with
    the soaking water
1 tsp cinnamon
1 tsp coconut oil
2 Tbl hemp seeds
1" vanilla bean

Combine in blender or Vita Mix.

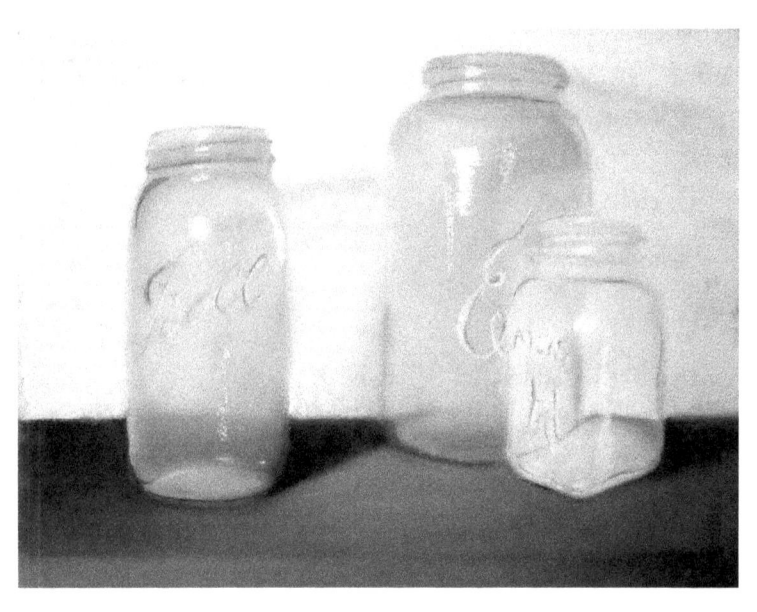

SPREADS, SAUCES, SPICES & CONDIMENTS

marinated red onions

1 large red onion
¼ cup olive oil
1Tbl balsamic vinegar

Slice red onion into 1/8" slices. Combine olive oil and vinegar and pour over onions in a bowl. Marinate for 1 hour.

Put on Teflex sheet and dehydrate for 12 hours at 110 degrees. They will still be moist when done.

homemade horseradish

½ cup chopped fresh horseradish root
1 date
filtered water to blend

Blend in a blended or food processor until a spreadable paste is made. It is very good on Nut & Veggie Burgers.

jalapeno relish

1 red bell pepper, chopped
3 jalapenos, diced
1 shallot, chopped
2 Tbl lemon juice
2 dates, soaked
salt and cracked black pepper to taste

Place all ingredients in a food processor and pulse a few times to desired consistency.

sweet relish

2 cups chopped cucumbers
1 cup chopped jicama
2 Tbl yellow onion
½ red bell pepper
¼ tsp ground ginger
1 tsp cinnamon
1 tsp curry powder
3 Tbl agave nectar

Pulse all ingredients in a food processor until the consistency of relish. Let marinate for at least 6 hours in fridge. Good on Nut & Veggie Burgers.

tomato-pineapple-green apple salsa

1 large tomato, finely chopped
1 cup fresh pineapple, finely diced
1 granny smith apple, finely diced
1 bunch cilantro, finely chopped
1 shallot, finely chopped
1 lime, juiced
Dash lime zest
1 clove garlic, minced
1 tsp sea salt

Combine all ingredients in a bowl. Add additional salt if necessary.

pickled beets

8 medium beets, sliced thin

1 lemon, juiced
dash salt
1 garlic clove, minced
5 dates, soaked
½ cup date soaking water
2 tsp whole pickling spices

Combine all ingredients except beets. Add beets to pickling mixture. Let marinate in fridge for at least 1 day. Store in refrigerator.

pico de gallo

2 large tomatoes, diced
2 jalapeños, chopped fine
1 onion, chopped fine
½ cucumber, chopped fine
2 avocados, chopped fine
¼ cup chopped cilantro
juice from 1 lime
2 tsp olive oil
sea salt and cracked black pepper to taste

pesto

Makes approx. 3 cups

2 cups packed fresh basil
¼ cup pine nuts
¼ cup walnuts
¼ cup pistachios
2/3 cup olive oil
1 Tbl minced garlic
Juice of 2-3 lemons
1 tsp salt (or more to taste)

Combine all ingredients in a food processor using the "S" blade. Add more salt to taste if desired. Excellent served over zucchini noodles or whole grain cooked noodles.

nut & sun-dried tomato pate

1 cup walnuts, soaked overnight
½ cup pumpkin seeds, soaked overnight
¼ cup sun-dried tomatoes, soaked overnight
¼ tsp dried thyme
½ tsp dried rosemary
1 Tbl herbs de province
½ tsp Herbamare
pepper to taste

Combine in food processor using the "S" blade until it forms a pate consistency.

sun-dried olive tepanade

1 cup sun-dried olives
2 cups walnuts, soaked overnight and drained
juice of 1 lemon
1/3 cup olive oil
1 Tbl miso
3 stalks celery, finely chopped
2 Tbl parsley, finely chopped

Combine all ingredients in a food processor.
Serve with crackers or on cucumber rounds.

vegetable pate

2 cups assorted veggies and/or sprouts
½ cup walnuts
2 Tbl nama shoyu
2 Tbl oil (can be olive, walnut, sesame, hazelnut, etc.)

Combine in food processor until creamy. You
can use a little water if necessary. This is a good
way to use leftover veggies.

marinara sauce

8 roma tomatoes
2 garlic cloves
1 shallot, diced
¼ cup parsley, chopped
1 cup basil
1 Tbl fresh oregano
sea salt and cracked black pepper to taste

Combine in food processor until smooth. Serve over zucchini noodles made with a Spirulizer or use as a dipping sauce for crackers or vegetables.

simple pasta sauce

1 cup sliced mushrooms
olive oil
dash salt

½ cup sun-dried tomatoes w/soaking water
1 cup chopped tomatoes
¼ cup fresh basil
¼ cup pine nuts

¼ cup chopped olives

Pour oil and salt over mushrooms. Let sit at room temperature for 1-2 hours. Dehydrate for 4-6 hours.

Combine sun-dried tomatoes, tomato, basil and pine nuts in food processor. Serve over zucchini noodles, whole-grain noodles, etc. Top with chopped olives.

rosemary gravy

¼ cup raw almond butter
2 Tbl white miso
1 garlic clove
½ red bell pepper
1 Tbl mince parsley
½ tsp dried or 1 ½ Tbl fresh rosemary
cracked black pepper

Put all ingredients in a blender and add purified water until it becomes gravy-like. Serve over nut loaves, etc.

baba ganoush

1 large eggplant
2 Tbl Tahini
¼ cup lemon juice
2 garlic cloves
¼ tsp salt
fresh cracked pepper
2 tsp olive oil
2 Tbl scallions, thinly sliced
2 Tbl fresh parsley, finely chopped
water to blend

Slice eggplant into ½" slices. Salt and set aside for about ½ hour. Rinse, dehydrate for about 2 hours at 100 degrees.

Place dehydrated eggplant along with Tahini, lemon juice, garlic and pepper in a food processor and blend using the "S" blade until smooth. Place in a bowl and drizzle with olive oil and tilt to that it covers the top. Sprinkle with scallions and parsley.

hummus

2 cups sprouted chick peas (sprout 2 days)
¾ cup olive oil
juice of 2 lemons
2 cloves garlic
¼ cup chopped parsley
2/3 cup Tahini
½ tsp sea salt
dash paprika

Put all ingredients in a food processor and blend using the "S" blade until smooth. Serve with carrot/celery/red pepper strips or on crackers.

almond hummus

1 cup almonds, soaked overnight and drained
¼ cup parsley, chopped
1 cup sesame seeds, soaked 6 hours
4 Tbl. lemon juice
2 Tbl. olive oil
2 tsp. cumin
½ tsp sea salt
1 garlic clove, minced

Blend in food processor. Serve with raw
crackers or sliced carrots/and or celery.

tahini dip

juice of 1 lemon
2 cloves garlic
2 Tbl agave
½ cup Tahini
2 Tbl tamari

Combine all ingredients in a blender and blend until creamy. Good for spring rolls, shushi, veggies, etc.

pizza appetizers

Any crisp cracker recipe

Toppings:

Seed cheese
Chopped olives
Sliced cherry tomatoes
Chopped basil
Drizzle with olive oil
Sprinkle with cracked black pepper

chard roll appetizers

Chard leaves
Cream cheese
Raisins
Pine nuts

Cut middle vein out of chard leaves. Place
cream cheese, raisins and pine nuts up the
center of the chard leaves and roll up. Serve as
an appetizer or a side dish.

dolmas

14 grape vine leaves in brine

4 chard leaves
2 cloves garlic
1 Tbl. red onion, chopped
½ cup chopped raw mild cheddar cheese
½ cup pine nuts
½ cup raisins
¼ cup olive oil
juice of 1 lemon
6 pitted calamara olives
salt & pepper to taste

Blend all but grape vine leaves in food processor until ground, but not mushy.
Put about 2Tbl of filling in each leave and roll up.
Cover with olive oil and refrigerate until firm and ready to serve.

non-fried beans

1 cup walnuts
1/3 cup pine nuts
1/3 cup almonds (soaked for at least 4 hours and drained)
1/3 cup sunflower seeds almonds (soaked for at least 4 hours and drained)
5 sun-dried olives
1/3 red bell pepper, chopped
½ cup olive oil
¼ cup water
1 tsp paprika
1 tsp cumin powder
½ tsp onion powder
¼ tsp or more cayenne (opt)
Celtic sea salt to taste

Process the nuts in a food processor until ground fine. Add remaining ingredients and process until creamy. This is so good on the spinach tortillas with tomatoes and avocado. It is very filling.

basic seed cheese

1 cup cashews
½ cup pine nuts
1 clove garlic
1 Tbl chopped shallot
herbs of choice
1 tsp white miso

Combine all of the ingredients in a blender with enough water to create a thick cream. Pour into a nut bag or cheesecloth and squeeze out the liquid.

Allow to ferment 3 hours. Store in fridge. Use the leftover liquid for dressings, sauces, etc.

cashew cream cheese

2 cups soaked cashews
½ cup raw macadamia nuts
½ cup lemon juice
¼ cup Rejuvalac* or miso & 1/8 cup water
2 tsp Nama shoyu (may use tamari or soy sauce)
1 garlic clove (small)
cracked black pepper

Combine in food processor using the "S" blade until very creamy. Store in the fridge.

*Rejuvalac is a drink made from soaking 1/2 cup wheat overnight, draining, then sprouting for 2 days (or until little white tails appear). At that time, cover with 4 cups purified water and let sit in a warm place until the liquid starts to have little bubbles and a slight lemon smell (about 12 hours).

cashew mayonnaise

1 cup cashews - soaked, drained and rinsed
2 Tbl lemon juice
¼ clove garlic
½ tsp nama shoyu
3 Tbl almond milk
½ tsp Herbamare

Combine in food processor using the "S" blade until very creamy.

cashew or pine nut cream

1 cup pine nuts or cashews, soaked overnight
  and drained
2 Tbl hemp seeds
2 Tbl maple syrup
1 tsp vanilla
Dash salt
Water as needed

Place nuts, hemp seeds, maple syrup & vanilla in blender. Add water to make a thick cream. Use as a topping for fruit.

candied sweet pecans

1 cup raw pecans, soaked overnight and drained
¼ cup date soaking water
1 Tbl mesquite powder
dash salt
dash cinnamon

Place soaked pecans in a bowl and add
remaining ingredients. Let marinate for 2 hours.
Dehydrate for 8 hours at 105 degrees.

spicy pumpkin seeds

1 cup raw pumpkin seeds, soaked overnight and
    drained
1/3 cup water from soaking dates (dates that
    have been soaking for at least 2 days)*
1 Tbl mesquite powder (opt)
1 tsp cracked red pepper
½ tsp salt

Combine date soaking water, mesquite powder,
cracked red pepper and salt.

Pour marinade over pumpkin seeds and
marinate 1 hour. Dehydrate for 24 hours or until
crunchy.

*you can substitute agave nectar or honey for
date soaking water.

pralines

1 cup pecans, soaked for about 4 hours and
    drained
8 dates, soaked overnight
1 Tbl raw honey

Combine dates and honey in food processor and
blend until creamy. Add date soaking water if
necessary to blend. Pour over pecans in a bowl.
Dehydrate for 12 hours. Serve as a topping for
ice cream or decorate desserts.

chocolate syrup

1 cup agave nectar
2 Tbl hazelnut oil
1 Tbl vanilla extract
1 cup ground cacao
dash salt

Blend in blender until smooth

almond flour

1 cup almonds, soaked overnight and drained

Dehydrate almonds about 12 hours. Put in food processor and grind as fine as possible (but not until it makes almond butter). Spread on Teflex sheet and dehydrate again until dry (about 6-8 hours).

spice blends

Za'atar (middle eastern)

1/8 cup sumac berries
1 Tbl dried thyme
1 Tbl marjoram
1 Tbl oregano
½ tsp salt
1 Tbl sesame seeds

Oriental

2 Tbl sesame seeds
1 Tbl dried garlic granules
1 Tbl dried minced onion
1/8 tsp cracked black pepper
1 tsp dried celery
1/8 tsp dried lemon peel
1 tsp mustard seed
1/8 tsp ground ginger

Mexican

6 Tbl chili powder
1 tsp onion powder
2 ½ Tbl ground cumin
1 tsp garlic granules
¼ tsp dried thyme
1 Tbl dried basil
1 tsp oregano
½ tsp black pepper

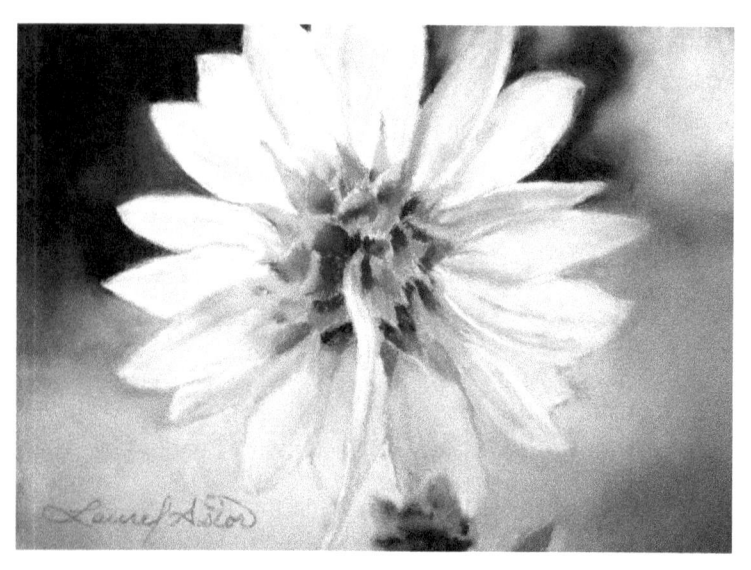

CRACKERS, BREADS & TORTILLAS

health-nut crackers

about 30 crackers

½ cup almonds, soaked overnight and
drained
½ cup sunflower seeds, soaked overnight
and drained
¼ cup sesame seeds, soaked overnight and
drained
½ apple, cored and shredded
1 stalk celery, chopped
¼ cup fresh parsley, chopped
¼ cup flax meal
2 Tbl lemon juice
2 Tbl dried spices/seasonings or 1 cup fresh
approximately 2 tsp. salt

Shred the apples in the food processor. Remove
and grind the almonds and seeds in the food
processor until finely ground. Add remaining
ingredients along with 1 cup of purified water and
the shredded apple. Place on a two dehydrator
trays using a Teflex sheet, scoring where you
want to break the crackers, and dry for about 12
hours. Remove the Teflex sheet and dry another
12 hours or until crisp. Store in a cool dry place.

flax caraway crackers

2 cups flax seed meal
2 cups water
1 apple, grated
1 cup walnuts, ground
1 Tbl caraway seeds
1 Tbl of your favorite seasoning
Sprinkling of Gamasio

Soak the flaxseed meal in the water for a few
hours. Add the rest of the ingredients, except
Gamasio, and stir until well mixed. Spread on a
dehydrator sheet and sprinkle with Gamasio. Dry
for 12 hours. Flip over and dry another 12 hours.
Store in a cool dry place.

pumpkin sesame crackers

½ cup pumpkin seeds, soaked overnight, drained
½ cup almonds, soaked overnight and drained
½ cup sunflower seeds, soaked overnight and
    drained
½ cup sesame seeds, soaked overnight and
    drained
1 stalk celery, chopped
¼ apple, grated
juice of 1 small lemon
6 sun-dried olives
½ cup flaxmeal
1 ½ Tbl vegetable seasoning
½ tsp sea salt
¾ cup purified water

Shred the apples in the food processor. Remove
and grind the almonds and seeds using the "S"
blade until finely ground. Add remaining
ingredients along with 1 cup of purified water and
the shredded apple. Place on a dehydrator tray
using a Teflex sheet and dry for about 12 hours.
Removed the Teflex sheet and dry another 12
hours or until crisp. Store in a cool dry place.

nut meal crackers

3 cups nut pulp from making nut milk
1 carrot, diced
2 stalks celery, diced
1 small shallot, diced
5 dates, soaked
1 ½ cups purified water (or date soaking water)
2 Tbl your favorite seasoning
1 tsp garlic powder

1 cup flaxmeal

Combine everything except flaxmeal in food
processor using the "S" blade. Blend well. Pour
into a bowl and add flaxmeal and stir well to mix.

Dehydrate for 12 hours – flip over – dry another
12-24 hours or until done. They will be more like
corn bread consistency than crackers. Very
good with soup and salad.

spinach tortillas

2 carrots, cut small
1 clove garlic
4 cups spinach leaves, chopped
1 Tbl dried onion
1 small shallot, diced
dash salt
1 cup cilantro, chopped
1 cup water
juice from 1 lemon
1 cup flaxmeal

Combine all ingredients except flaxmeal in food processor and blend using the "S" blade. Place in a bowl and add flaxmeal. Stir to mix.

Spread on Teflex sheets in 5 inch rounds and dehydrate about 8 hours or until dry, but still bends.

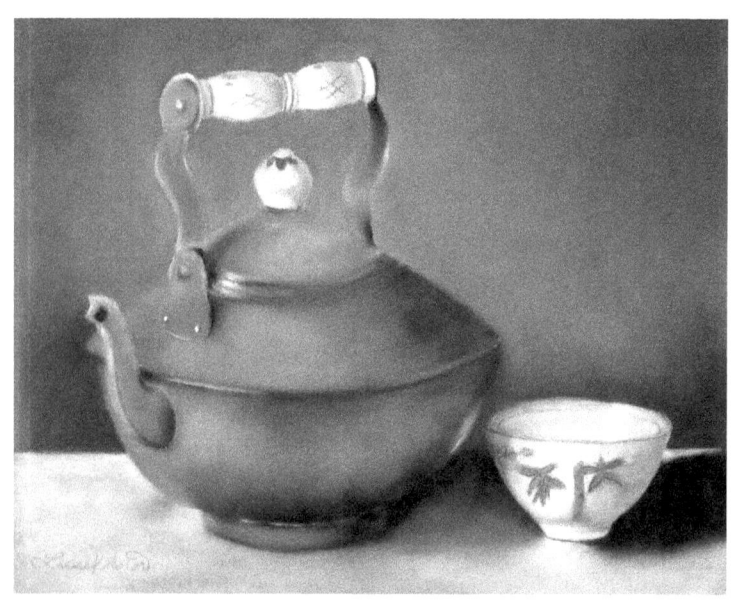

SOUPS

gazpacho

Serves 4

3 large tomatoes
2 cucumbers
1 red bell pepper
1 small jalapeno or cayenne (opt)
2 green onions
½ cup chopped cilantro
½ cup chopped parsley
1 clove garlic
3 Tbl olive oil
juice of 2 lemons
1 tsp cumin
1 tsp sea salt

Blend in food processor adding purified water as needed to reach desired consistency. Garnish with avocados, cilantro, and/or parsley.

creamy cauliflower dill soup

Serves 2

1 small head cauliflower
1 stalk celery, chopped
1 cup almonds, soaked overnight in 2 cups water

4 Tbl fresh dill
Herbamere to taste
2 Tbl white miso
Cracked black pepper
2 tsp olive oil

Rinse almonds and blend with 2 cups fresh water. Blend until frothy. Put remaining ingredients in blender with almond "milk" and blend until creamy. Serve with a sprig of fresh dill, and serve with dehydrated crackers crumbled and sprinkled over the top if you have any on hand.

creamy squash soup

Serves 4

3 cups butternut squash, steamed and cut into
   chunks
1 tsp nutmeg
1 cup cashews, soaked 2 hours and drained
½ fresh pear
1 stalk celery, cut into chunks
4 dates, soaked overnight
3 cups purified water
½ tsp sea salt
curry powder

Blend all ingredients in a blender until creamy.
Top with a light sprinkling of curry powder.

chinese vegetable soup

Serves 4

2 cups nappa cabbage
2 Tbl white miso
2 stalks celery, chopped
2 Tbl Nama Shoyu
2 carrots, chopped
2 tsp oriental seasoning
3 green onions, sliced
2 cups mung bean sprouts
4 dates, soaked in 1 cup water
½ cup fresh corn
   (save water)
6 snow peas, sliced in quarters

Combine cabbage, celery, carrots, green onions, dates & the 1 cup soak water, miso, Braggs, and oriental seasoning in a blender along with 1 cup purified water. Pour the liquid into a bowl. If you're using store-bought mung bean sprouts, slice them into 1" pieces, otherwise add whole sprouts, corn and snow peas to the liquid in the bowl (do not blend). Stir well. Garnish with a sprig of green onion.

corn chowder I

Serves 4

3 cups fresh corn kernels
1 small shallot, chopped
¼ tsp cardamom
3 cups homemade almond milk
1 tsp Herbamare
1 Tbl chopped fresh oregano
¼ tsp sea salt
cracked black pepper

Combine everything except corn in blender and blend until smooth. Stir in corn (don't blend) and serve. Garnish with chopped parsley or cilantro if desired.

People who do not typically like raw food will more than likely love this soup.

corn chowder II

Serves 2

2 cups almond milk
fresh corn kernels from 2 cobs
2 Tbl shallot, chopped
1 ½ Tbl cumin
dash Nama Shoyu
¼ tsp sea salt
cracked black pepper
1 avocado, chopped small
¼ bell pepper, chopped small
1 cup frozen peas, thawed

Combine almond milk, all but ¼ cup corn kernels, cumin, nama shoyu, salt and pepper in blender until frothy. Add avocado, bell pepper, and peas and stir (don't blend).

tomato soup

Serves 2

3 tomatoes, chopped
1 cup sun-dried tomatoes, soaked at least 4
   hours (save water)
2 cups tomato soaking water and additional
   water if needed
1 stalk celery with leaves, chopped
1 Tbl dried basil, or ¼ cup fresh, chopped
1 Tbl lemon juice
2 Tbl white miso
1 tsp cumin powder
1 Tbl olive oil
½ tsp garlic powder
1 tsp Herbamare
Garnish:
Fresh parsley, cilantro, celery seeds and
   pumpkin seeds (opt.)

Combine all ingredients in a blended and blend
until smooth and creamy. Garnish with chopped
parsley and cilantro and a sprinkling of celery
seeds and ground pumpkin seeds, if desired.

creamy celery soup

Serves 2

2 cups fresh celery juice
2 cups homemade almond milk
1 Tbl olive oil
5 sun-dried or regular olives
3 Tbl white miso
1 tsp celery seed
cracked black pepper to taste

Blend all ingredients in a blender until smooth.
Garnish with additional diced olives and a celery
leaf if desired.

hearty bean soup

1 cup cooked black eye peas
1 cup cooked adzuki beans
1 Tbl olive oil
1 large tomato
3 cups carrot/celery juice
½ cup sun-dried tomatoes, soaked and drained
(save water to use if necessary)
½ tsp garlic powder
1 Tbl fresh thyme
½ - 1 cup purified water (you can use tomato
    water)
sea salt to taste

Place peas, beans, olive oil, juices, tomatoes,
sun-dried tomatoes, garlic powder, thyme and
water in a blender. Add water to desired
consistency and blend until creamy.

☐

green curry soup

2 young green coconuts – meat & milk
1 Tbl grated lemongrass
1 Tbl lime juice
¼ cup cilantro, chopped
1" piece ginger, finely chopped
¼ cup basil, chopped
1 tsp umeboshi plum paste
2 Tbl olive oil
1 tsp roasted sesame oil
½ tsp curry powder
1 Tbl diced shallot
1 shredded carrot
1 Tbl green pepper, diced
½ cup cauliflower, cut small
¼ cup sliced almonds
1 cup chopped bean sprouts

Process coconut meat and milk with lemongrass, lime juice, cilantro, ginger, basil, umeboshi plum paste, olive oil, sesame oil curry powder and shallot in food processor. Add remaining ingredients and stir well.

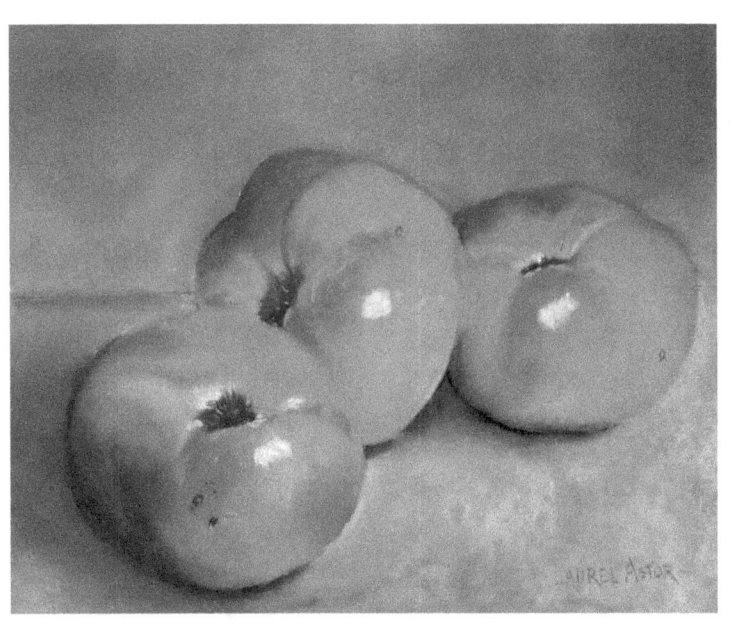

SALADS
&
DRESSINGS

chopped salad

Serves 4

2 cups pecans, soaked for one hour
2 carrots, chopped
2 stalks celery, chopped
2 c ups parsley, chopped
½ red bell pepper, chopped
3 Tbl fresh dill
Creamy Tahini Dressing

Put all ingredients except dressing in a food processor and pulse using the "S" blade just until chunky. Top with Creamy Tahini Dressing, and if desired, a dash of Eden's Seaweed Gomasio Seasoning. Serve on a bed of lettuce.

healing salad

3 cups chopped romaine lettuce
1 head chopped Italian parsley
2 sprigs mint, chopped
2 cups chopped whole tomatoes, or halved
cherry tomatoes
¼ cup sunflower seeds
juice from a large lemon

Toss all ingredients in a bowl. This salad is very
simple, but surprisingly delicious and healing. I
have served it as a main meal at times.

lentil and cumin salad

Serves 4

2 cups sprouted lentils
1 cup corn, fresh or frozen (thawed)
1 cup jicama, chopped
2 Tbl parsley
¼ cup red bell pepper, diced
juice from 1 lemon
2 Tbl olive oil
2 tsp cumin powder

Combine and serve on a bed of lettuce

marinated kale salad

Serves 4

5 cups finely shredded kale
2 Tbl sesame seeds
¼ cup olive oil
1 clove garlic, minced
1 Tbl lemon juice
½ tsp sea salt
10 sun-dried olives, chopped

Combine and let marinate overnight in the fridge.

You can substitute chard for kale. Kale has a
high amount of calcium.

sprout salad

Serves 4

1 cup mung bean sprouts
1 cup sprouted sunflower seeds
¼ cup sprouted quinoa
1 carrot, sliced
1 red pepper, chopped
1 tomato, chopped
½ cup cured olives, chopped
2 Tbl pine nuts
1 avocado, cut in chunks
2 Tbl lemon juice
1 cup cilantro, chopped
1 cup parsley, chopped
1 tsp dried or 1 Tbl fresh dill
½ cup dressing of your choice

Mix and serve on a bed of lettuce.

adzuki & wild rice salad

Serves 4

1 cup adzuki beans, sprouted 3 days
1 cup wild rice, sprouted 2 days
3 cups shredded kale
3 Tbl olive oil
2 cloves garlic
1 cup fresh or frozen peas
cracked black pepper
1 tsp fresh thyme
sea salt to taste

Combine all ingredients and serve. Will hold well
in the fridge.

sweet & sour lentils

Serves 2

2 cups sprouted lentils
1 carrot, diced
1 apple, shredded
2 tsp olive oil
1 tsp ginger, grated
1 tomato, diced
1 small shallot, finely diced
2 Tbl Nama Shoyu
1 clove garlic, minced

Combine all ingredients in a bowl and serve on a bed of lettuce or as a side dish.

thai mango salad

Serves 2

2 mangos, chopped
¼ cup chopped raw peanuts
1/3 cup chopped cilantro
2 green onions, chopped
1 clove garlic, minced
1/3 cup shredded coconut
4 dates, soaked and mashed
juice of 1 lime
1 tsp Nama Shoyu

Mix together lime, shoyu and dates in a small bowl. Place remaining ingredients in a large bowl and toss with lime sauce. Serve on a bed of lettuce.

chinese salad

salad:
2 cups store-bought mung bean sprouts
3 green onions, sliced thin
½ cup thinly sliced bok choy
½ cup diced red bell pepper
1 cup small broccoli flowerettes
¼ cup sliced raw almonds
1 cup finely shredded purple cabbage
¼ cup unhulled sesame seeds
6 sugar snap peas, sliced 1"
1 jalapeno, diced small on the diagonal

sauce:
½ cup cold-pressed sesame oil (not roasted)
1 Tbl nama shoyu
½ tsp lemon juice
4 dates, soaked

Combine salad ingredients in a large bowl.
Combine sauce ingredients in blender and blend
until creamy. Pour sauce over salad. Mix well
and serve.

indian cabbage salad

4 cups shredded cabbage
1 carrot, grated
½ red bell pepper, cut into small chunks
½ cup grated coconut
½ cup chopped raw peanuts
½ cup bottled, Indian-style Mango Chutney
6 dates, soaked overnight (use water)
juice from 1 lemon
½ tsp ground cumin
½ tsp ground brown mustard seed
salt to taste

Combine first 5 ingredients in a large bowl. Combine chutney, dates, soaking water, lemon juice, cumin, mustard seed and salt. Pour chutney mixture over cabbage mixture and mix well. This is a variation of a recipe by Rhio. People who haven't tried raw food love this salad.

wild rice & pea salad

Serves 2

1 cup cooked wild rice, cooled
½ cup peas, fresh or frozen
½ cup raw cheese, cubed small
½ cup carrots, chopped small
¼ cup red or orange bell pepper, chopped small
2 crimini mushrooms, chopped small
2 Tbl olive oil
Salt and pepper to taste

Cook rice and cool either to room temp or in
fridge. Add the remaining ingredients and stir.

tabouli

1 cup cooked quinoa
1 Tbl dried lemon balm
1 bunch parsley, chopped very small
1 finely chopped tomato
5 green onions, sliced very thin
1 large lemon, juiced
¼ to ½ cup olive oil
¼ cup almonds, soaked overnight and chopped
½ cucumber, chopped small
sea salt and cracked black pepper to taste

Cook quinoa. Cool. Add the rest of the ingredients and mix well being careful not to break apart the quinoa. Stays good in fridge for at least 4 days.

greek salad

Serves 2

1 head Romaine lettuce
3 radishes, sliced
3 green onions, sliced
1 cucumber, sliced
1 red pepper, diced
10 sun-dried or Calamata olives
10 cherry tomatoes, halved
½ cup shredded raw cheese
¼ cup olive oil
juice of 1 lemon
1 Tbl chopped fresh oregano
sea salt and cracked black pepper to taste

Combine all ingredients in a bowl and mix well.

sea salad

Serves 2

¼ cup Wakame sea vegetable
¼ cup diced red bell pepper
¼ cup orange juice
½ cup diced jicama
1 Tbl sesame seeds
sea salt to taste

Combine Wakame and orange juice and allow to
sit long enough for the Wakame to become soft.
Add the remaining ingredients and stir.

papaya salad

Serves 2

2 papayas, chopped
2 dates, chopped
¼ tsp freshly grated ginger
dash freshly grated nutmeg

Combine and top with coconut sprinkles if desired.

coleslaw

½ head cabbage, sliced very thin
1 carrot, grated
¼ cup + 1 Tbl agave nectar
3 Tbl cider vinegar
½ cup Vegannaise
1 tsp sea salt
1 tsp celery seeds
cracked black pepper to taste

Place cabbage and carrots in a bowl. Whisk agave, vinegar, Vegannaise, salt, and celery seeds until blended. Pour over cabbage and mix well.

basil salad

Serves 2

5 leaves Romaine lettuce, sliced into ¼" pieces
½ cup chopped tomatoes
10 chopped olives
¼ cup chopped cucumber
½ avocado, chopped
¼ cup fresh basil dressing (p.116)
½ cup honey mustard dressing (p.117)
2 Tbl hemp seeds

Toss well and season with sea salt and cracked black pepper to taste. Top with hemp seeds.

"tuna" salad

½ cup almonds, soaked overnight and drained
1 cup walnuts, soaked 4 hours and drained
1 Tbl lemon juice
1 Tbl nama shoyu
2 tsp kelp powder
1 chopped shallot
½ cup finely diced celery

Place all ingredients except celery into food processor and pulse until the consistency of tuna. Place in bowl and mix with celery.

Serve atop Natures Path Manna Bread that has been dehydrated for about 2-3 hours, crackers, vegetables, or a bed of lettuce. You can also spread Cashew Mayonnaise, homemade Sweet Relish, or whatever you like on the bread before topping with tuna salad.

red bell pepper, carrot & seaweed salad

1 red bell pepper, diced small
2 carrots, shredded
1/2 cup soaked seaweeds of choice
1 tsp agave nectar
1 tsp balsamic vinegar
1 Tbl roasted sesame oil
1 Tbl sesame seeds

Combine red bell pepper, carrots and seaweed in bowl. In a separate bowl combine remaining ingredients and pour over veggies.

dilled green beans

3 cups fresh green beans, cut in half
½ cup jicama, sliced in 2" pieces
1 small shallot, minced
¼ cup sliced almonds
¼ cup finely chopped fresh dill
1 Tbl. olive oil
2 tsp lemon juice
Herbamare to taste

Let marinate in fridge a few hours before serving.

basic salad dressing

¼ cup vinegar
2 cloves garlic
1 Tbl Dijon mustard
½ cup olive oil
2 Tbl chopped parsley

Blend in the blender until creamy. You can add
fresh herbs, fruits, olives, fresh juices, sesame
seed, agave, honey, etc. for different flavors.

creamy tahini dressing

approx. ½ pint

½ cup olive oil
juice of 3 lemons
2 Tbl white miso
¼ cup Tahini
8 dates, soaked
cracked black pepper

Combine all ingredients in a blender. Add
enough purified water to make a creamy
dressing.

You may add vegetable seasoning, orange juice,
etc. to make different flavored dressings. This is
my favorite dressing.

french dressing

approx. ¾ pint

½ cup olive oil
4 dates, soaked
¼ cup orange juice
juice of ½ lemon
¼ tsp ground mustard powder
¼ tsp Herbamare
sea salt and cracked black pepper to taste

Combine in a blender until smooth. This is a
sweet dressing.

dilly dressing

approx. ½ pint

½ cup rejuvalac*
2 Tbl lemon juice
½ cup olive oil
¼ cup chopped dill
2 Tbl cashew mayonnaise
2 tsp Herbamare
cracked black pepper to taste

Combine in blender until creamy.

*Rejuvalac is a drink made from soaking 1/2 cup wheat overnight, draining, then sprouting for 2 days (or until little white tails appear). At that time, cover with 4 cups purified water and let sit in a warm place until the liquid starts to have little bubbles and a slight lemon smell (about 12 hours). Strain and keep in fridge.

fresh basil dressing

½ cup olive oil
1 Tbl walnut oil
¼ cup walnuts
2 Tbl chopped shallots
1 cup fresh basil
1 tsp Dijon mustard
1 tsp agave nectar

Combine all ingredients in blender until creamy. This dressing will get a little thick after being refrigerated, but if you put it on top of greens and mix it in, it will loosen up.

honey mustard dressing

1 quart

2 Tbl brown mustard seeds
1 Tbl hemp seeds
¾ cup cider vinegar
10 Tbl stone ground prepared mustard
1 ½ cups raw honey
1 tsp garlic salt
1 clove garlic
1 cup canola oil
½ cup unroasted sesame oil

Place all ingredients except oils in a blender. Blend until mixed. Mix canola and sesame oil together. Add oil in a steady stream until fully blended. Let blend for a couple more minutes after adding all of the oils. This is so good you will want to eat it by the spoonful when you first make it.

sesame dressing

approx. 1 pint

1 ½ cups olive oil
½ cup cider vinegar
4 Tbl. sesame seeds
3 Tbl agave nectar
2 Tbl frozen orange juice concentrate
2 tsp your favorite seasoning
1 clove garlic
2 Tbl nama shoyu
cracked black pepper to taste

Combine all ingredients in a blender and blend until creamy.

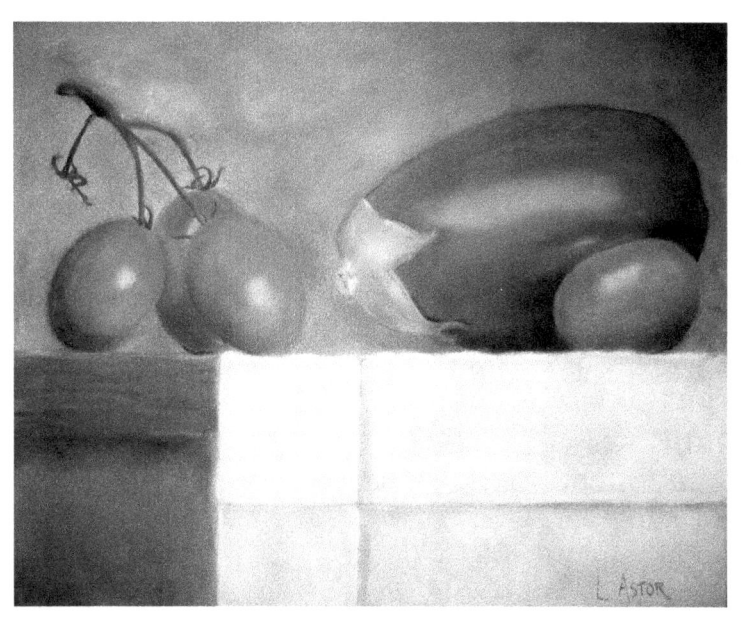

ENTREES

spaghetti

sauce:

1 large tomato	1 small leek
1 red bell pepper	1 cup fresh basil

½ cup sun-dried tomatoes, soaked for at
 least four hours (or longer)
½ cup pine nuts or walnuts, soaked at least
 four hours (or longer)
juice of ½ lemon
Italian seasonings to taste
salt to taste

zucchini made into thin spaghetti noodles using a spiralizer.

topping:
1 avocado, chopped
fresh basil leaves
additional pine nuts for topping

Combine the sauce ingredients (including sun dried tomato soaking water) in a food processor using the "S" blade. Spoon sauce over zucchini noodles and top with fresh avocado chunks, chopped basil leaves, and pine nuts.

This is my favorite entrée. It is a good recipe to make for people when introducing them to raw food.

nut & veggie burgers

8 patties

½ cup almonds soaked overnight & drained
½ cup sunflower seeds soaked overnight &
   drained
1 cup sesame seeds
1 small shallot, chopped
1 red bell pepper, chopped
1 zucchini, chopped
1 carrot, chopped
½ cup packed fresh basil leaves
2 Tbl olive oil
2 Tbl fresh parsley, chopped
1 Tbl lemon juice
1 tsp your favorite seasoning
½ tsp vegetable seasoning of your choice

Blend all ingredients in a food processor with just
enough water to hold mixture together.
Dehydrate for 24 hours – turn and dehydrate
another 6 or 7 hours. Serve on lettuce leaf with
thick slices of tomato, avocado and Creamy
Tahini Dressing. May add sun-dried olives,
Marinated Onions, Sweet Relish and Homemade
Horseradish Dressing if desired.

You can make a large batch of these and they
will last about a week in the fridge.

nut loaves

Serves 4

1 cup sunflower seeds, soaked overnight
and drained
1 cup sesame seeds, soaked overnight and
drained
1 cup pumpkin seeds, soaked overnight and
drained
¼ cup chopped fresh chives
3 cups carrot pulp (from juicing)
1 tsp vegetable seasoning of your choice
1 tsp salt
½ cup flaxmeal
enough water (approx. 1 cup) to hold it
together

Combine all ingredients in a food processor.
Make into 5" x 3" loaves and dehydrate for about
8 hours.

If you have a dehydrator that can accommodate
large loaves, you can make one big loaf. Serve
when it is warm out of the dehydrator.

Very good with Rosemary Gravy.

romaine roll-ups

Mexican:
1 avocado, diced
½ tomato, diced
½ carrot, shredded
12 sun-dried olives, sliced
3 Tbl red bell pepper, diced
¼ tsp cumin
sea salt to taste

Oriental:
½ carrot, shredded
2 green onions, diced
3 Tbl red bell pepper, diced
6 snow peas, sliced into 1/8" pieces
Nama Shoyu, to taste
2 Tbl seawed, soaked

Roll in Romaine leaves and serve right away.

romaine rolls
Serves 4

4 large romaine leaves

filling:
1 carrot, shredded
1 beet, shredded
8 arugula leaves (or sliced kale)
8 Tbl raw Cream Cheese
12 small sprigs of fresh dill
8 Tbl marinated red onion
4 large fresh basil leaves (or equivalent)
4 Tbl spicy pumpkin seeds
dash Nama Shoyu in each leaf

Fill each of the leaves with 4 equal parts of each item in the filling list. Roll up and hold together with plastic wrap until ready to serve.

rice patties

Serves 2

1 cup wild rice, sprouted
dash Nama Shoyu
1 cup diced mushrooms
2 green onions, diced
1 Tbl chopped fresh parsley
1 carrot, diced small
1 lemon, juiced
cracked black pepper (opt.)
1 tsp your favorite seasoning
1 clove garlic, minced
1 Tbl fresh thyme

Put everything except rice into a food processor
and process using the "S" blade. Put into a bowl
and add the rice. Make into patties and dehydrate
12 hours.

zucchini pasta
w/cream sauce

Serves 4

sauce:
1 cup pine nuts
juice of 2 lemons
1 clove garlic
½ tsp herb seasoning to taste
1 tsp white miso

3 zucchinis, spiralized

Combine sauce ingredients in a food processor using the "S" blade until creamy.

Put the zucchini through a garnishing machine (spiralizor) to create angel hair-like pasta threads.

Pour sauce over zucchini and serve. You can garnish with additional pine nuts, if desired.

veggies with peanut sauce

sauce:
3 Tbl raw peanut butter
2/3 cup purified water
1 clove garlic, minced
2 dates, soaked
dash cayenne pepper or red pepper flakes
1 Tbl lemon juice
seas salt to taste

veggies:
You can use any amount of a variety of veggies.
The following are some examples

Sliced cabbage   Green beans
Celery, sliced thin   Beets, diced
Carrots, julienned   Bean sprouts
Avocado slices to decorate

Combine sauce ingredients in a blender. Blend until smooth.

Put veggies in separate piles on a large serving plate. Pour sauce over veggies and serve.

spring rolls

You can use any or all of the below ingredients for the spring roll filling:

carrots, cut into matchsticks
fresh basil
napa cabbage, shredded
fresh cilantro
green onions, cut into matchsticks
red cabbage, shredded
mung beans, cut in half
jicama, cut into matchsticks
beets, cut into matchsticks
red bell pepper, sliced thin
avocado, sliced

large spring roll shells made with rice (these are not raw)

You can purchase them from oriental markets. They also come made with tapioca flour. If you prefer to use all raw ingredients, slice cucumbers very thin, overlap them to make a square and roll up with filling ingredients.

dipping sauce for Spring Rolls:

½ cup Tahini, 4 dates (or 1 tsp. maple syrup or agave) - soaked, 2 tsp nama shoyu, 1 garlic clove, 1" piece of ginger and enough water to make the sauce creamy and smooth.

Soak spring roll shells in water for just a minute (until slightly soft). Place on cutting board, fill with about 1 cup of various filling ingredients and roll up, tucking in the sides as you go.

Blend ingredients for the dipping sauce in food processor using the "S" blade. Dip rolls in dipping sauce.

enchiladas

Serves 2

4 spinach tortillas

2 cups corn, cut from cob
2 tsp cumin
1 shallot, minced
4 Tbl raw salsa of your choice
8 Tbl raw Cream Cheese
1 sliced avocado
¼ cup chopped cilantro
2 Tbl chopped sun-dried olives

Additional salsa and sliced avocado

Combine corn and cumin and mix well. Divide ingredients into quarters and layer ¼ on one half of each tortilla shell. Fold over and cover with additional salsa and sliced avocado.

stuffed tomatoes

serves 4

2 large tomatoes

4 Tbl olive oil
1 cup spinach, chopped
½ cup pine nuts or sunflower seeds
½ cup fresh basil, chopped
1 avocado, diced small

Hollow out tomatoes. Dice the tomato that you remove and add to remaining ingredients. Stuff tomatoes with mixture and serve.

rice casserole

Serves 4

1 cup cooked wild rice (1/2 cup dried)
1 onion, finely chopped
2 garlic cloves, minced
1 ½ cup finely chopped mushrooms
1 large tomato, finely chopped
¼ cup chopped sun-dried tomatoes, soaked for
    at least 2 hours
¼ cup golden raisins
¼ cup finely chopped parsley
¼ cup finely chopped walnuts
2 Tbl olive oil
dash salt
cracked black pepper

Combine ingredients and serve immediately.
Can put in fridge and eat as a cold salad also.

chickpeas & mango

Serves 4

1 Tbl olive oil
1 tsp ground cumin
1 large onion, finely diced
1 tsp garam masala
4 garlic cloves, minced
1 tsp ground turmeric
2 small green chilies, sliced
3 large tomatoes, diced
1 tsp ground coriander
4 large dates, soaked overnight

2 Tbl chopped cilantro
2 Tbl shredded mint
1 cup cooked chickpeas
1 large mango, peeled and diced

Combine first 10 ingredients. Let sit for a couple of hours or overnight in fridge.

Add remaining ingredients and mix well.

mushroom & zucchini quesadeas w/fresh salsa

Serves 2

4 sprouted grain tortilla shells
½ large zucchini, sliced thin
6 mushrooms, any kind
½ bell pepper, sliced thin
½ lb. grated raw cheese

Layer veggies and cheese atop 1 tortilla and cover with another one. Heat gently until cheese melts.

Salsa:
4 tomatoes, chopped small
½ bell pepper
1 lime, juiced
1 Tbl onion, chopped small
½ cup finely chopped cilantro
1/3 cup chopped sun-dried tomato, soaked for
    at least 4 hours
dash vinegar
salt to taste

Combine all salsa ingredients and serve with quesadeas.

almost raw spaghetti

Serves 4

Sauce:
3 medium tomatoes, chopped
1/8 cup onions, chopped
½ bell pepper, chopped
1 cup fresh basil
½ cup sun-dried tomatoes, soaked at least 4 hours (use soaking water)
1/3 cup walnuts
1/3 cup pistachios or pine nuts
dash red wine
½ tsp Italian seasoning
dash Nama Shoyu

Combine first 11 ingredients in food processor and blend until just slightly chunky.

½ grated carrot
½ grated zucchini

Cooked artichoke flour noodles.

Place noodles on plate. Layer with carrot and zucchini and top with sauce.

coconut green curry delight

Serves 2

Meat from one young green coconut, cut into ¼ inch strips (make sure you have one that has meat at least 1/8" thick)
½ cup diakon radish, julienned then cut into 2" pieces
¼ cup shredded carrot
½ cup asst. exotic mushrooms, sliced then
1 Tbl. nama shoyu
1 Tbl. rice wine vinegar
1 Tbl. olive oil
¼ cup snap peas, cut into ½" pieces
¼ cup red bell pepper, julienned then cut into 2" pieces
1 green onion, sliced thin
¼ cup cilantro, chopped
¼ cup basil, chopped

Topping:
1 Tbl. chopped raw peanuts
¼ tsp black sesame seeds

Curry:

¼ cup coconut milk
2 Tbl. rice wine vinegar
¼ cup olive oil
1 tsp. Umeboshi plum paste
1 tsp. Thai Kitchen Fish Sauce
1 Tbl. fresh grated lemongrass or 1 tsp dried
2 Tbl. agave nectar
1" piece ginger, chopped fine
1 Tbl. toasted sesame oil
1 tsp Thai Kitchen Green Curry Paste

Place mushrooms in a bowl and add the 1 Tbl nama shoyu, 1 Tbl rice wine vinegar and 1 Tbl olive oil. Mix well and place on Teflex sheet and dehydrate for 4-6 hours.

Combine curry ingredients in a bowl and mix well. Put in fridge for a couple of hours for the flavors to blend.

Combine diakon radish, carrot, mushrooms, snap peas, bell pepper, green onion, cilantro and basil in a large bowl. Mix well. Add coconut strips and stir in being careful not to break them. Divide into two and place each portion on a serving plate. Pour half of the curry sauce onto each serving and top with peanuts and sesame seeds. Num.

avo sandwiches

4 pieces Natures Path Manna Bread
1 avocado, sliced
½ tomato, sliced thin
4 slices raw cheddar cheese
2 Tbl raw spaghetti sauce or salsa
Cashew Mayonnaise
Greens and/or sprouts

Spread Cashew Mayonnaise and Spaghetti
Sauce or Salsa on 2 slices of Manna Bread (may
dehydrate for a few hours to warm). Top with
remaining ingredients. Top with remaining 2
slices of bread and serve.

extremely yummy enchiladas

Raw spinach tortillas
Cream cheese
Spinach
Olives, sliced
Avocado, sliced
Pico de Gallo
Tomatoes, chopped

Fill tortillas with a layer of cashew cheese, spinach, olives, avocado, Pico de Gallo and tomatoes. Top with additional Pico de Gallo.

tamales with raw mole
Serves 4

12 corn husks
Soak in warm water until pliable.

Tamale mixture:
12 ears corn, cut from cob
1 cup walnuts
1 Tbl cumin
1 tsp sea salt
½ tsp coriander
1 cup cashews, soaked for 4 hours, drained

Combine in food processor until smooth.

Mole:
1 shallot, diced
1 Tbl walnut or olive oil
¼ tsp coriander
½ tsp anise
1 Tbl chili powder
1 tsp agave
1 Tbl pumpkin seeds
½ tsp cinnamon
2 Tbl ground cacao
1 Tbl raw almond butter
1 Tbl raisins

Mole continued:

1 garlic clove
1 Tbl sun-dried tomatoes (soaked overnight –
  save water)
Tomato soaking water plus enough water to
  make 1 cup

Sesame seeds
Pica de Gallo
Cashew cream cheese

Roll tamale mixture in husks. Dehydrate 4 hours
or longer. Remove from husks just prior to
serving and cover with mole sauce. You may top
with pica de Gallo and cream cheese. Top with
sesame seeds.

avocado boats

Serves 2

1 avocado cut in half
½ tomato, diced
½ cup "tuna salad"
1 Tbl cucumber relish
1 Tbl Cashew Mayonnaise
Hemp seeds

Scoop avocado meat out of each half. Cut into chunks. Combine with the rest of the ingredients and fill empty avocado shell with mixture. Sprinkle with hemp seeds.

mushroom, cheese & tomato fettuccini

Serves 2

1 yellow summer squash
approx. ¼ tsp salt
2 Tbl. olive oil
½ cup cherry tomatoes
½ cup chopped raw sharp cheddar cheese
1 cup assorted mushrooms, chopped
1 tsp. balsamic vinegar
1 tsp nama shoyu
1 Tbl. fresh rosemary leaves
2 Tbl. chopped fresh oregano
1 Tbl minced shallot or red onion

Using a spiralizer, make squash into fettuccini style noodles. Sprinkle with salt and let sit for a few hours. Place tomatoes in a small bowl; add 1 Tbl olive oil, salt and pepper. Place on dehydrator tray. Using the same bowl put mushrooms, vinegar, nama shoyu and rosemary in and mix well. Place on another dehydrator tray and dehydrate both tomatoes and mushrooms for about 8 hours. Place squash, mushrooms, tomatoes, oregano and red onion in a bowl and mix until well blended. Divide in half and serve in bowls.

ceviche

1 pound fresh sashimi grade salmon (not frozen), chopped into small bite-size chunks

1 pound fresh shrimp (not frozen), cut in small pieces

5 limes, juiced (or to cover fish)

½ bunch cilantro, chopped

3 Tbl chopped shallot, chopped fine

1 avocado, chunked

½ cup cherry tomatoes, cut in half

1/3 cup cider vinegar

1/3 cup raw blue agave nectar or honey

½ cup raw mild cheddar cheese, chopped small

Celtic sea salt

Place salmon and shrimp in a bowl and salt with Celtic sea salt. Pour in lime juice mixing to coat, and marinate all day or overnight in fridge. Combine cilantro, shallot, avocado, tomatoes, cheese, vinegar and agave to blend flavors. Add to fish and stir carefully as not to break up salmon. Add Celtic sea salt to taste.

luscious romaine wraps

½ pound sushi grade tuna, sliced
3 limes (or to cover tuna)

½ recipe spring roll dipping sauce
2 oz. extra sharp raw cheese, sliced
½ cup grated carrots
½ cup grated beets
½ cup grated diakon radish
1 avocado, sliced

8 large romaine leaves

Marinate tuna in lime overnight. Pour off lime
juice. Roll romaine leaves with tuna, dipping
sauce, cheese, carrots, beets, radish & avocado.

asian coconut noodle salad

meat from 4 young green coconuts, sliced into
    matchstick noodles
½ cup raw peanuts, chopped
2 radishes (diakon or red) diced
3" cucumber, diced
¼ cup sprouted mung beans
¼ cup fresh basil, chopped
¼ cup fresh cilantro, chopped

Peanut sauce:
¼ cup coconut water
1 Tbl raw blue agave nectar
4 Tbl organic roasted chunky peanut butter

Celtic sea salt
Sesame seeds

Combine coconut water, agave, and peanut
butter to blend.

Place coconut meat, peanuts, radishes,
cucumber, mung bean sprouts, basil and cilantro
in a bowl. Pour peanut sauce over top, and salt
to taste and stir to blend. Top with sesame
seeds.

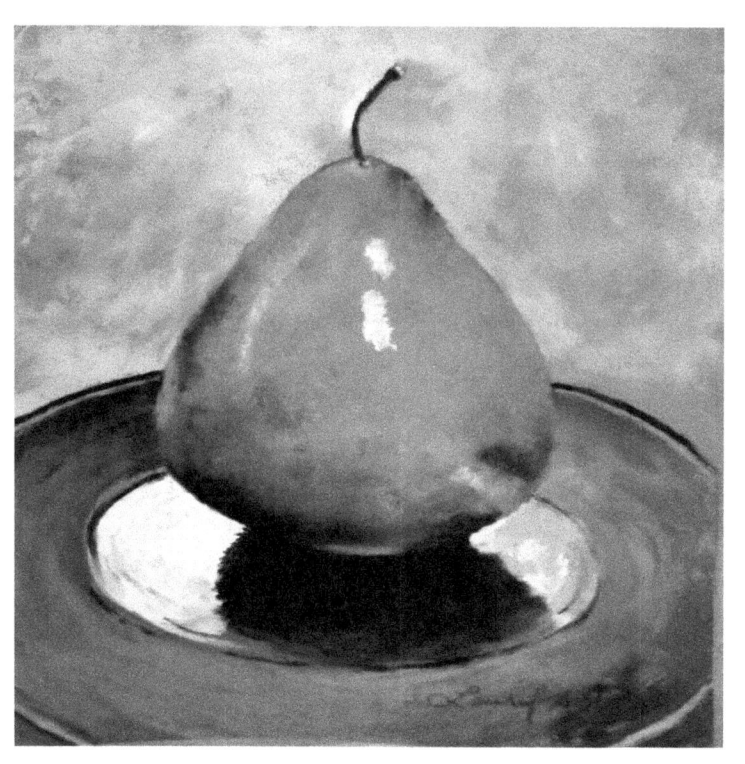

DESSERTS

chocolate fudge
rolled in coconut

2 cups walnuts
1 cup raisins
2 Tbl cocoa powder
4 dates, soaked
dash cinnamon
shredded coconut

Grind walnuts in a food processor using the "S" blade until finely ground. Add raisins, cocoa powder, dates and cinnamon.

Shape into 2" logs and roll in coconut.

cacaoballs

1 cup Raw Honey
1 cup coconut oil
1 cup cacao powder
dash Celtic sea salt
Cacao nibs
Hemp seeds
Chopped pecans

Place bottle of coconut oil in warm water to soften. Combine all ingredients in a bowl and stir well. Place in fridge until it just starts to stiffen. Remove from fridge and make into 2" balls. Roll in cacao nibs, chopped pecans and/or hemp seeds.

You can roll these in anything you like. Some suggestions are chopped nuts, powdered cacao, cayenne, shredded coconut, sesame seed or get creative!

These are my favorite sweet treats. I usually eat one a day. Make sure to use creamy raw honey or it just won't hold together.

mango cream mousse

1 cup pecans, soaked overnight and drained
½ cup macadamia nuts, soaked overnight and
　　drained
½ cup cashews, soaked overnight and drained
12 dates, soaked at least 2 days (save juice)
½ cup date soaking water
2 ripe mangos
4 Tbl coconut oil
1 tsp vanilla

Place jar of coconut oil in hot water to liquefy.

Place all ingredient in a food processor and
blend using the "S" blade until it is the
consistency of cream.　Put in parfait or wine
glasses and top with grated coconut.　Refrigerate
until set.

cherry coconut cream

1 cup cashews, soaked and drained
1 cup golden raisins, soaked (save water)
1 tsp vanilla
2 cups fresh sweet cherries
½ cup shredded coconut

Put all ingredients in a food processor, including the raisin water. Blend using the "S" blade until creamy.

You may use this in parfaits, to top fruit, or as a dip for fruit. You can also place in the freezer, and when ready to serve, let thaw just a bit and blend in the food processor and serve as ice cream.

mango parfait

½ cup raw mixed nuts (almonds, hazel nuts,
     cashews, pecans, walnuts, or whatever you
     have on hand)
6 dates, soaked
1 banana, sliced very thin
1 mango
shredded coconut

Blend nuts in a food processor using the "S"
blade until finely ground. Add dates and a small
amount of date soaking water until nuts start to
hold together.

In burgunder wine glasses (or parfait glasses)
put a layer of the nut mixture, then a layer of the
sliced bananas.

Place peeled and pitted mango in a food
processor and blend until creamy. Pour atop the
bananas.   Sprinkle with shredded coconut.

vanilla ice cream

2 ½ cups almond milk or raw milk
1 cup maple syrup
1 tsp pure vanilla extract
dash salt

Stir together and process in ice cream maker.

strawberry ice cream

1 pint strawberries
1 cup maple syrup
2 ½ cups almond milk or raw milk
1 tsp pure vanilla extract
dash salt

Slice strawberries into a bowl. Pour maple syrup
over the strawberries and marinate for 1 hour.
Mash about ½ of the strawberries.

Add the almond milk, vanilla and salt. Stir.

Process in ice cream maker or pour into ice cube
trays, freeze, then blend in food processor until
creamy, or process in ice cream maker.

chocomint ice cream

1 recipe vanilla ice cream
½ cup cacao nibs
2 drops peppermint essential oil
Mix together and process in ice cream maker.

gelato

Chocolate

2 cups cashews, soaked for 3 hours
1 cup maple syrup
2 Tbl ground cacao

Mocha

2 cups cashews, soaked for 3 hours
1 cup maple syrup
2 Tbl ground cacao
2 Tbl instant coffee

Mango

1 mango, chopped
2 cups soaked cashews
1 cup dates, soaked overnight

Blend in food processor until creamy. Freeze for at least 8 hours in covered container. Scoop out with ice cream scoop into small bowl.

prune whip

1 ¼ cup pitted prunes
¼ cup freshly squeezed orange juice
½ cup cashews, soaked 2 hours and drained
4 dates, soaked overnight (save water)

Combine all ingredients in a blender and blend until creamy. Add a little of the date soaking water if necessary. Serve in small wine glasses and garnish with a mint sprig.

energy bars

1 apple, shredded
1 cup pecans, soaked overnight and drained
1 cup almonds, soaked overnight and drained
2 cups sunflower seeds, soaked overnight and
   drained
1 cup sesame seeds, soaked overnight and
   drained
1 cup raisins, soaked in 2 cups purified water
(save water)
5 black mission figs, soaked
1 cup dates, soaked (save water for other uses)
1 tsp cinnamon
1 tsp sea salt
1 cup shredded coconut
1 cup flaxmeal

Shred apple by hand, or use a food processor.
Put in a large bowl. Process pecans, almonds,
sunflower seeds and sesame seeds in a food
processor using the "S" blade. Add to shredded
apple. Combine raisins, figs, cherries, dates,
cinnamon & salt using the "S" blade. Add to nut-
apple mixture. Add flaxmeal and coconut and
mix well. Dehydrate for 6 hours. Turn over and
dehydrate 6 more hours.

sesame nut bars

1 ½ cup dates, soaked overnight
½ cup sesame seeds
½ cup cashew pieces
½ cup pumpkin seeds
2 Tbl honey

Combine in food processor by pulsing. Keep some of it chunky. Dehydrate for 8 hours.

fiery coffee balls

1 cup cashews
1 cup walnuts
2 Tbl instant organic coffee (dry)
Small pinch dried ground habanaro
1 cup dates
2 Tbl ground cacao

Process in food processor. Make into balls and roll in cocao powder.

almond macaroons

2 cups shredded coconut
6 dates, soaked overnight
½ cup coconut oil
½ cup agave nectar
½ tsp vanilla
1 cup almonds, soaked overnight and drained
dash salt

Process dates, coconut oil, agave, vanilla and almonds in a food processor. Place in a bowl and add coconut. Mix well. Using a small melon scoop, place balls on Teflex sheets and dehydrate 12 hours, remove Teflex and dehydrate another 12 hours.

chocolate candy

8 Tbl coconut butter
1 cup cacao powder
1 Tbl raw agave nectar
½ tsp vanilla extract

Put in fridge until hard. Form into a log – put back in fridge until hard again. Slice into ½" slices. Keep cold and eat fast.

sweet lime pie

crust:
2 cups pecans
1 cup dates
dash cinnamon
3 dates, soaked

filling:
juice from 5 limes*
1 cup cashews, soaked and drained
2 cups dates, soaked and drained
¼ cup coconut oil

Place pecans in a food processor and blend using the "S" blade until pecans are broken into very small pieces. Add dates and cinnamon and blend until dates are ground. Add soaked dates and blend until mixture starts to bind together. Press into a 9" pie plate.

Combine the filling ingredients in the food processor and blend until smooth. Add just a little water if it doesn't blend well. Pour into crust and let set in fridge for at least 2 hours.

*May substitute 3 lemons for the limes.

chocolate pecan pie

crust:

½ cup walnuts
½ cup almonds
1 cup raisins

2 Tbl cocoa powder
dash cinnamon
5 dates, soake

filling:

1 cup pecans, chopped
3 bananas, sliced

topping:

2 cups dates, soaked
juice of ½ orange
dash nutmeg

Combine walnuts, almonds, raisins, cocoa powder, and cinnamon in a food processor using the "S" blade until finely ground. Add dates and continue to blend until mixture holds together. Press into glass pie plate.

Pulse pecans in a food processor using the "S" blade until chopped. Pour into crust. Put sliced bananas on top of pecans.

For filling, combine dates, orange juice and nutmeg. Blend until creamy. Refrigerate for at least 1 hour.

berry pie

crust:

1 cup almonds	8 dates
1 cup pecans	dash cinnamon

filling:
2 cups fresh or frozen (thawed) raspberries,
blueberries, blackberries, or strawberries
2 cups cashews, soaked and drained
6 dates, soaked at least 2 days (save water)
date soaking water

topping:
2 large bananas, sliced
slivered almonds
1 Tbl coconut

Combine crust ingredients in a food processor
using the "S" blade. Press into a 9" pie plats.

Combine filling ingredients in the food processor
with just enough date soaking water to make
creamy. Pour into crust.

Top with bananas, almonds and coconut. Chill
for at least 2 hours to set.

german chocolate pie

Nut Crumble Crust:

½ cup shredded coconut   ½ cup date sugar
1 cup pecans   ½ cup raisins

Combine in food processor until crumbly.

Chocolate Filling

1 cup Antonio Peuo's ground chocolate
1 cup cashews, soaked for 4 hours
2 Tbl coconut butter
1 tsp vanilla extract
dash salt

Combine in food processor until creamy.

Topping:

½ recipe Pralines, chopped
¼ cup shredded coconut

In a springform pan, press nut crumble crust into bottom
with a small lip. (Can use a pie pan also). Fill with
chocolate filling and top with pralines and coconut. Press
the pralines and coconut slightly into the filling to adhere.
Refrigerate for at least 2 hours. Yum.

cheesy blueberry tart

crust:
1 cup dates
1 cup almond flour
3 dates, soaked

filling:
1 cup cashew cheese recipe made without the
    nama shoyu, garlic and pepper
½ cup agave nectar or raw honey
2 Tbl coconut oil

topping:
1 cup fresh blueberries
8 dates, soaked
2 Tbl coconut oil
dash salt

Combine dates and almond pulp flour for the crust in food processor using the "S" blade. Process until finely chopped. Add soaked dates and process until it starts to bind together.

Combine ingredients in food processor (no need to wash the processor in between) and process until very creamy. Let sit in fridge until set. You may put in the freezer to set quicker.

Once the filling has set, combine the topping ingredients in the food processor and process until pureed. Top the filling with the blueberry puree and put in fridge to complete set all layers.

Decorate with blueberries and candied pecans, if desired.

cheezecake
with raspberry cream
glaze

crust:

1 cup walnuts	dash salt
1 cup almonds	1 cup raisins
dash cinnamon	2 dates, soaked

cream cheese filling:
2 cups cashews, soaked and drained
½ cup maple syrup
½ cup coconut oil

glaze:

¼ cup coconut oil	4 dates, soaked
½ cup macadamia nuts	dash salt
½ cup fresh raspberries*	½ tsp vanilla
2 Tbl maple syrup	

Before starting place the jar of coconut oil in a bowl of hot water to liquefy.

For the crust - combine walnuts, almonds, cinnamon and salt in a food processor and process using the "S" blade until finely ground. Add raisins and process until they are ground. Add dates and process until mixture starts to bind together. Press into spring form pan coming up on the sides about ½".

For the filling - combine all cream cheese filling ingredients in the food processor and blend until creamy. (There is no need to wash food processor between layers). Pour into crust and use a spoon to smooth out the top. Place in the fridge and let set until firm. This may take a couple of hours.

For the glaze - Combine all ingredients in the food processor and blend until creamy. Pour over the cream cheese filling and spread out being careful not to disturb the filling so that the pretty layers will show when you cut the cheesecake.

*May use strawberries, blueberries, or ½ cup orange juice in place of raspberries.

blueberry pie

Crust:

2 cups almond flour
½ cup dates
½ cup dried apricots

Filling:

2 cups cashews
2 cups blueberries
½ cup honey
¼ cup coconut oil
1 Tbl chocolate powder

Combine crust ingredients in a food processor.
Press into a 9" pie plate. Combine filling
ingredients in a food processor until blended.
Pour into crust.

pecan pie

Crust:

1 cup almonds
1 cup pecans
2 Tbl chocolate powder
½ cup dates
½ cup dried apricots
Dash cinnamon

Filling:

1 cup honey
2 Tbl coconut oil
Dash salt
1 cup whole pecans

Combine crust ingredients in a food processor. Press into a 9" pie plate. Combine honey, coconut oil and salt in a food processor until blended. Add pecans and stir (don't process). Pour into crust.

creamy & rich chocolate walnut torte

bottom layer:

2 cups walnuts

1 cup raisins

dash cinnamon

2 Tbl cocoa powder

4 dates, soaked

middle layer:

1 banana

1 cup dates, soaked

¼ tsp vanilla

topping:

½ cup ground walnuts

Bottom layer: put walnuts in food processor and grind using the "S" blade until fine. Add raisins, cinnamon & cocoa powder – blend. Add soaked dates and process until the mixture starts to ball up. Press into a spring form pan coming up about 1 inch on the side.

Middle layer: place banana, dates and vanilla in food process and blend until cream. Pour on top of bottom layer.

Topping: grind walnuts in food processor or coffee grinder and sprinkle on top.

peach blueberry crisp

Serves 2

Crisp
½ cup almond flour
½ cup rolled oats
2 Tbl walnut oil
4 Tbl maple syrup
¼ cup date sugar
dash salt

2 peaches, cut into chunks
¼ cup maple syrup
¼ cup fresh blueberries
dash salt

Topping
¼ recipe cashew cream

Combine crisp ingredients in a bowl. Dehydrate overnight or about 12 hours.

Place peaches in a bowl with the maple syrup and stir to coat well. Dehydrate 6-8 hours or until soft.

Divide peaches and blueberries into two bowls. Cover with crisp and top with cashew cream.

ambrosia cake

Crust:

1 cup walnuts	1 cup raisins
1 cup almonds	dash salt & cinnamon

Combine ingredients in a food processor and then press into a spring form pan.

1st Layer:
1 sliced mango
2 sliced white peaches
2 sliced bananas

2nd Layer:
1 cup cashews
1/3 cup coconut butter
1/3 cup maple syrup

Combine in food processor and layer atop fruit

3rd Layer:
1 cup fresh cherries, pits removed
¼ cup maple syrup
2 Tbl coconut butter
4 dates

Combine in food processor and pour over top. You can substitute the fruit with anything that is available.

This is my favorite dessert.

fruit chocolate tart

Crust:
½ cup pecans
5 macadamia nuts
Juice of one small orange or clementine
¾ cup dried coconut
¼ cup honey

Grind nuts in coffee grinder. Mix all ingredients in a small bowl. Spread on Teflex sheet (doesn't have to be perfect). Dehydrate for about 8 hours.

Layers:
#1
2 Tbl ground cacao
1/3 cup agave
½ cup coconut butter

Blend in food processor until creamy.

#2
½ cup cashews, soaked 4 hours
½ cup dates, soaked 4 hours
½ tsp vanilla
1 Tbl coconut butter

Blend in food processor until creamy.

#3
2 cups chopped fruit, such as strawberries, bananas, mango, peaches, etc.

Topping:

1 cup pitted cherries (or raspberries, blueberries, strawberries)
1/3 cup agave nectar
1 Tbl coconut butter

Blend in food processor until liquid.

Layer crust (can be in pieces), then #1, 2 & 3, then top with cherries sauce. Refrigerate for at least 4 hours.

cherry pecan cookies

1 cup golden raisins, soaked for about 1 hour
1 cup cashews, soaked for about 1 hour
1 cup flax meal
1 cup fresh pitted cherries
1 cup shredded coconut
¼ cup raw pecans
dash cinnamon
dash vanilla extract
dash almond extract

Combine in food processor and place flattened balls on Teflex sheet. Dehydrate for about 8-10 hours or until firm.

apricot fig cookies

½ cup dried apricots
½ cup dried figs
1 cup macadamia nuts
1 cup pecans
1 tsp vanilla

Combine in food processor and add a little water at a time as necessary to blend. Place flattened balls on a Teflex sheet and dehydrate for about 8-10 hours or until firm.

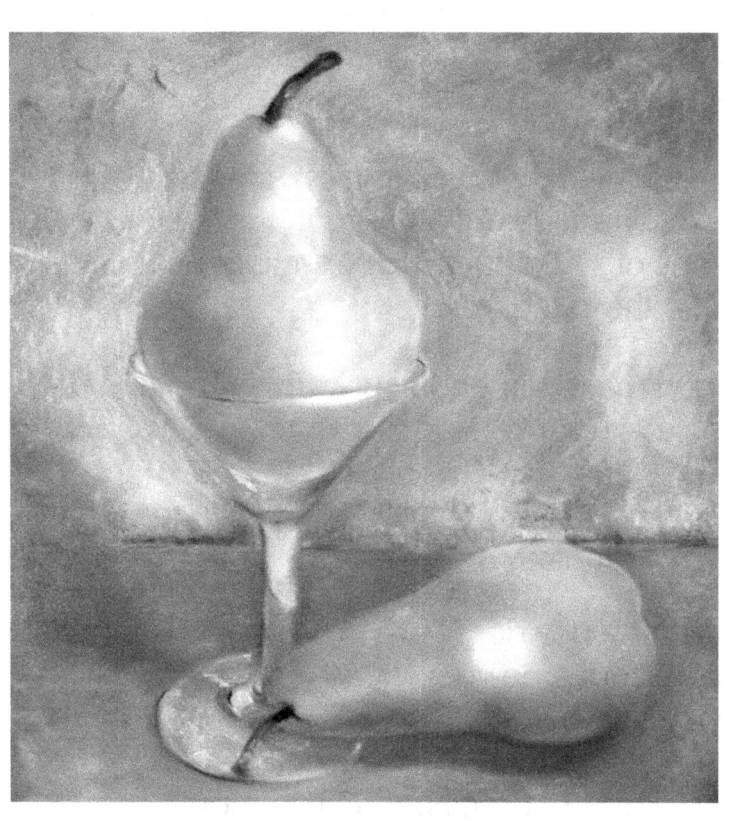

BEVERAGES

almond milk

Makes 1 quart

1 cup almonds, soaked overnight and drained*
1 quart purified water
6 dates or 1/3 cup raisins

Combine all ingredients in a blender and blend until frothy and liquefies. Strain through cheesecloth or a nut bag, collecting the liquid. Store in the refrigerator.

You can make almond flour with the pulp, or use it in salads, crackers, etc.

You can also add the following to make flavored milks:

3 Tbl cocoa powder
3 Tbl mesquite powder
3 fresh strawberries
1 fresh peach
2 tsp mixture of equal parts cinnamon,
   cardamom, cloves & nutmeg

Depending on the sweetness desired, you can add additional dates when blending.

*you may substitute other nuts

strawberry, peach, chocolate, goji berry shake

Serves 2

2 cups raw almond milk
8 cacao beans, ground in coffee grinder
½ stick cinnamon, ground in coffee grinder
¼ cup Goji berries
2 Tbl agave nectar, or to taste
4 strawberries
1 peach

Soak ground cacao and cinnamon in almond milk for at least ½ hour. Put almond milk with cacao and cinnamon along with the rest of the ingredients in a blender and blend until creamy.

watermelon cooler

Serves 4

10 cups diced watermelon
¼ cup canned coconut milk
¼ cup agave nectar

Blend in blender until creamy.

green tea chai

2 ½ cups seed milk made with ½ cup almonds, ½ cup pumpkin seeds, ½ cup soaked raisins (with soaking water) and 2 dates (use almond milk recipe for instructions)
3 tsp equal amounts ground cinnamon, cardamom, fenugreek, fennel, black pepper and anise
The contents of one green tea bag (any kind that you like)
6 additional dates

Blend in blender and let sit for about 20 minutes to let flavors blend. You can make this into an ice cream also.

Combine all ingredients in a blender. Serve with a celery stick.

aphrodisiac

2 cups almond milk
1 tsp maca powder
2 Tbl hemp seed
2 Tbl cacao nibs
4 Tbl agave
1 banana
4 strawberries
¼ cup blueberries
¼ cup raspberries

Blend in blender until creamy.

mocha frapaccino

Serves 2

2 cups almond milk (or other nut milk)
1 Tbl organic instant coffee
2 Tbl ground cacao or nibs
¼ cup agave nectar

Blend in a blender until creamy. Serve right
away with the froth bubbly on top.

bloody mary

2 cups fresh tomato juice
¼ cup fresh celery juice
1 tsp homemade horseradish (p. 27)
1 Tbl lemon juice
seasoning salt and cracked black pepper to taste

green smoothie

2 cups homemade Almond Milk
1 cup greens of your choice (young spring,
    romaine, arugula, spinach, etc.)
1 cup blueberries (fresh or frozen)
1 banana*
¼ cup Agave
1 Tbl green powder of your choice

Blend in blender until smooth.

*take bananas that are going soft - cut them up and put
them in the freezer for use in smoothies.

Index

Deliciously Raw will show you how to prepare meals that are incredibly delicious, healthy and beautiful. Raw food is fun, creative and interesting. Eating this way is very doable and brings vitality and energy, and maintains a body that is vibrant, trim and healthy.

This book is also about my personal journey of healing and discovery. I hope it will inspire you to venture into a new way of eating and living.

Laurel Astor
(970) 618-4627
laurelastor200@gmail.com